MW01032096

PRESENCE

PRESENCE

Published in 2021 by Hardie
Grant Books, an imprint of
Hardie Grant Publishing

Hardie Grant Books (London)
5th & 6th Floors
52–54 Southwark Street
London SE1 1UN

Hardie Grant Books (Melbourne)
Building 1, 658 Church Street
Richmond, Victoria 3121

hardiegrantbooks.com

British Library Cataloguing-in-
Publication Data. A catalogue
record for this book is available
from the British Library.

Presence
ISBN: 9781784883782

10 9 8 7 6 5 4 3 2 1

Publishing Director and
Commissioner: Kajal Mistry
Project Editor: Kate Burkett
Design: Claire Warner Studio
Illustrations: Evi O. Studio
Copy-editor: Tara O'Sullivan
Proofreader: Lucy Rose York
Indexer: Vanessa Bird

Colour reproduction by p2d
Printed and bound in China by
Leo Paper Products Ltd.

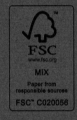

FSC
www.fsc.org
MIX
Paper from
responsible sources
FSC™ C020056

LISA LISTER

PRESENCE

KNOW YOURSELF
CLAIM YOUR POWER
TAKE UP SPACE

Hardie Grant

BOOKS

CONTENTS/

Part two:

CLAIM YOUR POWER /68

Part three:

TAKE UP SPACE /124

YOUR PRESENCE IS YOUR POWER /168

PRESENCE: A SELF-INVOCATION

PRESENCE:
A SELF-
INVOCATION

My presence is powerful. I'm a beacon
of mother-loving light. My body is a place
of creativity and power. I'm seen and
I shine. Bright.

I do not apologise for my appearance
and what I wear and how I style my hair.

I accept compliments with a big, open
heart. (And also know that I don't need
them in order to feel whole and complete.)

I know, trust, respect, honour and revere
my body, myself and my living experience.

I shine light into my dark places –
real and perceived – so that I can own
all my parts.

For sure, I've made mistakes. I've messed
up. I've failed. I'm human. I don't punish
myself for them, I acknowledge them,
learn from them and grow.

I refuse to accept labels of shame and
humiliation, of 'not worthy' and 'not
enough' that have been given to me
simply for being a woman in the world.

I shake myself free of the shackles of
'shoulds' and societal constructs and
dream, manifest and speak my life
and reality into being.

I DECLARE...

PRESENCE: A SELF-INVOCATION

I HAVE VALUE.

I AM **VITAL.**
I AM **RADIANT.**
I AM **SENSUAL.**
I AM **POWERFUL.**
I AM **IN PROCESS.**
I AM **IN PROGRESS.**
I AM **WHOLE.**

INTRODUCTION

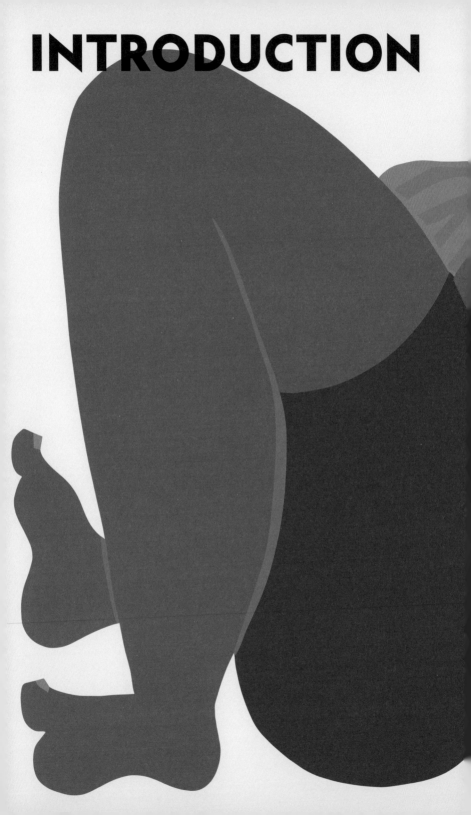

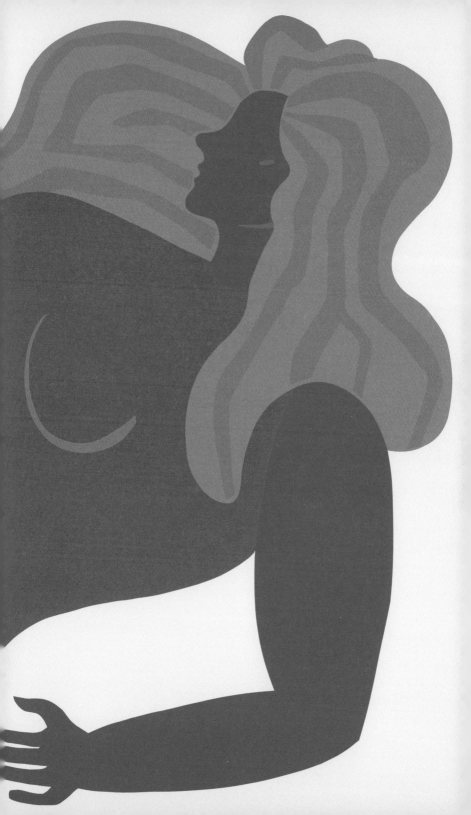

INTRODUCTION

Are you a woman who knows the power of her presence? A woman who nourishes, nurtures and prioritises her own wants, needs and desires? A woman who knows her value and worth? A woman who has a big heart and fierce boundaries? A woman who lifts and inspires others? A woman who can light up and captivate an entire room? A woman who doesn't look outside herself for approval and who, instead, validates herself and dares to shine?

Bright.

Really bloody bright.

I mean, that's the ideal scenario, right? To be THAT woman.

Except you, like me, may think it takes courage and wild strength to be THAT woman, because you, like me, have probably been taught from a very early age that, in order to 'show up' in the world, you need to do any – or all – of the following:

——— Fake it till you make it.

——— Meet totally unrealistic beauty expectations.

——— Feel bad when your perfectly fabulous-as-they-are skin/ thighs/hair/boobs do not meet said expectations, then go and buy ALL. THE. THINGS. that you're told will improve them.

——— Put on a persona based on the kind of person you *think* people want you to be.

——— Wear a variety of masks for different people, occasions and situations simply as a way to navigate a world that makes you feel less-than and not enough.

We're in a cycle of collective trauma simply by being women in a world of systems and structures that are not set up in our favour. Societal expectations like those described above can keep us in a consistent state of distrust and disconnect from ourselves, our bodies, each other and the world. This creates and supports the limiting beliefs, patterns and behaviours that we've been taught and told. Beliefs that have usually been implanted, subconsciously, to keep us feeling less-than, not worthy and in a state of constant comparison and competition with each other.

It's no surprise that many of the main recurring health problems and concerns that women experience are linked to chronic inflammation: a direct physical response to the long-term trauma, stress and anxiety that this sense of disconnect and distrust can cause in the body. Such conditions include, but are not limited to: chronic pain, disease, menstrual health problems, stress, burnout, anxiety and panic attacks. So, when asked to stay present, to reclaim our power, to reconnect with our bodies, to trust ourselves, to feel our feelings and to tend to our own needs, wants and desires, of course many women resist. We've forgotten who we were before we were told who to be. We no longer recognise ourselves, we have no point of reference for what it is that we need, want or desire because we're simply doing what we need to do in order to survive.

Which is why I'm writing this book.

To help you remember.

I want you to remember, in every way, that understanding, and being present to, the power of your own presence doesn't mean simply learning about body language, posture and how to wear a red lip (although I can totally help you with that; I do love a red lip). It's about self-discovery, reconnecting with your body, finding your true-to-you frequency and then aligning with it and amplifying it so that you no longer have to put on an act. It's not about makeovers or transformations, it's about flipping the switch on limiting beliefs and rewriting your story. A story where you trust yourself. A story where you honour and revere your body. A story where you recognise the instinctual felt truths in your heart and gut as your own innate wisdom. A story where you never shame, blame or abandon yourself again.

It's about owning who you are – *all* of you, the light and the dark parts – and knowing that, regardless of all the real or perceived mess-ups, failures and mistakes you've made (and the recognition that you *will* make more, because, y'know, you're human), you're still so bloody worthy of nourishment, nurturing, joy and big gorgeous, glorious love.

I want for you to be fiercely present to your own presence: to acknowledge, embrace and cultivate it.

Your own magnetic, radiant presence.

A presence that has not been faked to 'please' others, and is not a mask to hide behind.

A presence that is simply you: true, real and powerful, without apology.

This doesn't mean you have to be loud, bold and show-y (although you totally can be); it doesn't mean you have to dye your hair pink or get a full sleeve of tattoos (although you totally can); it simply means knowing and embracing the truth of who you are, and acknowledging that, in any given moment, it is subject to change. (In fact, *my* truest expression changes from one menstrual phase to another.) It's more about honouring yourself and respecting the ever-changing, oceanic, rhythmic nature of *your* creative power and expression, and having the self-love, self-respect and self-confidence to show up for yourself first and foremost, so that you can then show up for your family, for your community and for the planet.

This is the power of your presence.

And the act of becoming present to it, of cultivating it? That's self-love. Not *just* the 'have-a-bath-and-take-a-walk-in-nature' kind of self-love[1] that is often written off as *the* most overused phrase *ever* (I mean, let's face it: we've all given those social media posts the side-eye, right?), but potent self-care, the kind that involves being in honest and real connection with yourself, knowing what you need and making sure those needs are met because you KNOW you deserve it.

A woman who is in an active relationship with her body – a woman who is able to tend to, resource *and* nourish herself? Well, she's a game-changer and a paradigm-shifter.

Look, the last thing you need is another self-help manual, or an 'expert' telling you what to think and do. This *isn't* a 'how-to' book. It's not a replacement for therapy, either. I definitely won't be telling you how to 'solve' your problems or how to 'fix' anything.

This is an *'I've got you, we've got this, we're in it together – let's explore'* book, where I share insight, wisdom and guidance.

I've spent the last 15 plus years working with women and their bodies as a trained women's health practitioner, somatic embodiment coach, well woman therapist, yoga for bigger bodies teacher and menstrual maven. I'm also a woman in the world with my own lived experience of the fierce intelligence held in my body and I want, more than anything, to support you as you become present to the power of your own magnetic, captivating presence.

Everything I share in this book is an invitation to work and connect with *your* bodily state. Self-responsibility is most definitely required. Take what feels right and leave the rest.

How does that sound?

When you become present to the power of your presence, which, FYI, is a daily, life-long practice, you start to feel a reliable and consistent sense of connection to yourself, and to life.

You are able to navigate wisely from your body, and you are able to make smart decisions without looking outside yourself for someone else to fix or rescue you.

You trust yourself, and because of that, you're able to trust others and others trust you.

---

[1] I personally have big respect for this kind of self-love, but I'm aware that it often creates eye-rolls and can deter from the fact that, at its core, self-care is a daily act of showing up for yourself, tending to yourself, and nurturing and nourishing yourself and, well, that shit isn't always easy.

Your capacity for new possibilities and greater vitality and joy in your life grows.

You have more energy and feel more present, resourced and vital: you feel aligned.

Your relationships and self-expression have space to grow and bloom.

You feel fortified. You have strength, and it's from this place of strength and resilience that you're able to power up, show up, create and express what it is you came here for this lifetime.

Because honestly, if ever there was a time the world needed women to be aware and present to the power of their presence, to reconnect to their bodies, each other and the planet, to be seen *and* heard, to be self-sovereign, to make a difference and to lead – straight from the heart and gut – it's now.

WHEN YOU'RE A WOMAN WHO KNOWS THE POWER OF HER PRESENCE, YOU KNOW:

———— all the insidious games that are being played to keep you anxious, compliant and not nourished.

———— that you can shake free of the societal, cultural and familial shackles and show up for yourself, as yourself.

———— how to connect to your centre and fill yourself up in all the ways that feel right and good for you.

———— that when you're nourished and fecund, you're radiant and magnetic, and become a beacon of mother-loving light.

———— that you resonate at your own real-to-you frequency.

———— being you is a superpower.

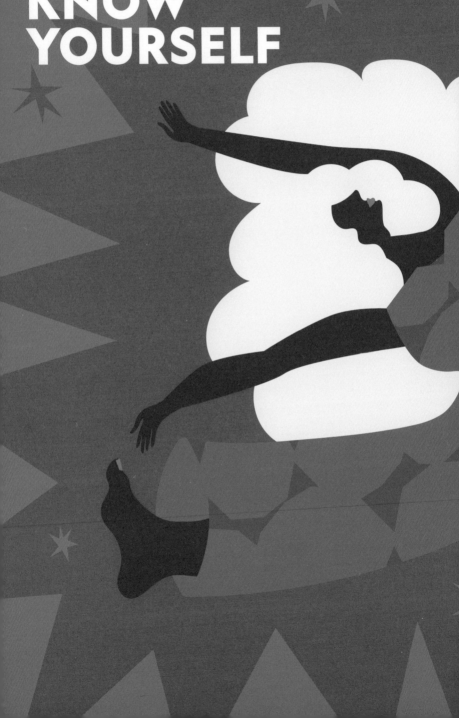

PART ONE: KNOW YOURSELF

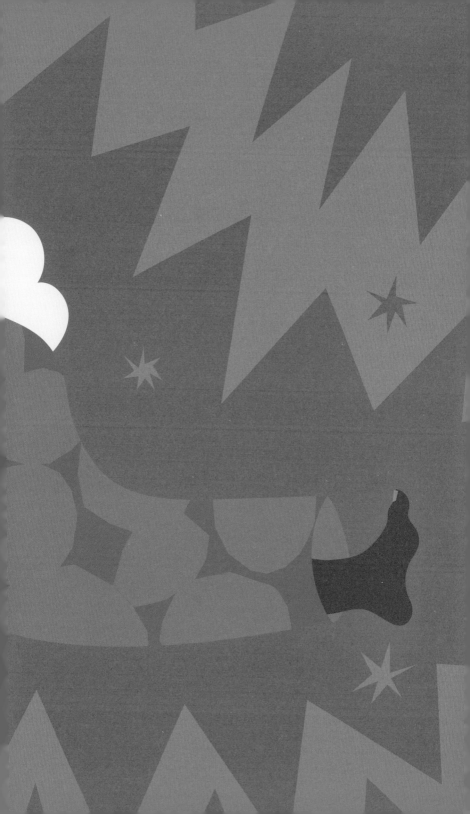

1: RECONNECT WITH –
AND LISTEN TO –
YOUR BODY

**(With big love
and a shit ton
of compassion)**

'Trust yourself.'
'Listen to your body.'
'The body never lies.'

Like so many deep and profound concepts that get made into social media posts and quoted without nuance and context, the thought of trusting yourself and listening to your body can feel like a really great idea in theory – but in reality?

Not so much.

If you feel in *any* way disconnected, disassociated and separate from your body, or if you experience anxiety, depression or panic attacks and your body doesn't feel like a safe space, then if you *did* listen to your body and you *did* always trust what it was telling you, there's a really good chance that you'd be aborting missions left and right, making poor decisions or making no decision at all. In order to be able to trust our bodies and have confidence in our gut feelings and intuition, we first need to be able to inhabit our bodies as a safe space that we feel connected to and comfortable in.

When you're not present in your body, you:

——— are unable to feel – physically, emotionally, spiritually;

——— are not able to feel the joy, pain, hope or fears of others;

——— find it hard to trust yourself and your intuition;

——— find it difficult to learn, change and transform;

——— fear being rejected;

——— feel you are not good enough;

——— compete with other women;

——— fear speaking up and/or being seen;

——— let others feel powerful at your own expense;

——— wait for permission and outside validation.

WHY DO WE ABANDON OURSELVES?

Oh, let me count the ways.

Technological overwhelm, pain (whether physical, emotional or spiritual), eighty-hour work weeks, social media competition and comparison, lack of in-real-life connection and community, trauma (whether personal, generational or societal), doing too much for too long, self-doubt, juggling a demanding job with being a good parent *and* a great lover, being *all* the things to *all* the people (except yourself, obvs) and… well, that's just for starters.

Many of us internalise negative experiences from early in childhood, whether they involve the criticism of others, or familial and societal beliefs. We experience certain feelings of shame, blame and humiliation simply for being women: for looking a certain way; for *not* looking a certain way; for not having the right skin tone or body shape; for menstruating; for not menstruating; for being 'too much' or 'not enough'. We berate ourselves for all the times we've wanted to say 'no' but didn't, and for all the times we've said 'yes' and wished we hadn't. And that's just the stuff from *this* life. We're also carrying whatever went down in our family lineage, too – and we're holding it *all* in our bodies. Add to that societal hypnosis and… well, is it any wonder we want to disconnect?

What is societal hypnosis?

Societal hypnosis comes from a series of small, seemingly inconsequential stories, actions and situations that have been slowly drip, drip, dripped into our psyches throughout our lives. These events rewire our neurology in a negative way, so that our bodies become conditioned to feel consistently fear-filled, not good enough, not worthy and unsafe.

This societal conditioning or hypnosis keeps us in a state of disconnection – from our true nature, from Mumma Nature, from our creativity, our rhythmic intelligence and from our cyclical connection to our bodies, the seasons, the moon and the cosmos.

It makes us question our relationships with *everything*.

YOU'RE NOT BROKEN.

IT'S SOCIETAL SYSTEMS AND STRUCTURES THAT ARE BROKEN.

It makes us think we're broken and not good enough. It gives us low self-worth and low self-esteem.

And when we think and feel like this, we are *far* easier to sell to and to manipulate. We're less likely to strive and thrive, create and be great, and to grow and really trust what we know. We assume that we're powerless.

When we are conditioned to think and feel in this way, it's much harder to trust ourselves. And when we don't trust ourselves, it's rare that our bodies feel like a safe place.

WHAT HAPPENS WHEN YOUR BODY DOESNT FEEL SAFE?

To exist in a body that doesn't feel safe in this world is really bloody painful.

So, we develop a survival strategy. Some of us cut.

Some of us over-eat. Some of us binge eat. Some of us don't eat at all.

Some of us become 'too busy' or distracted so that we don't have time to actually feel. We become self-destructive. Or we keep ourselves small and unseen. Or we don't allow ourselves the resources and nourishment we need in order to function, restore, grow and flourish.

When we're in this survival state, shitty things can start to happen to our bodies: pain, disease, discomfort, anxiety, depression, gnarly PMS and period-related disorders. These ailments send us a message, via the pain. They are telling us: *'Wake up, pay attention.'* Yet we rarely listen.

We don't know how.

No one told us how.

Instead, we think our bodies hate us.

We think they betray us.

So we shut down.

We switch off. We reject our own bodily feelings.

For many of us, our lives are so busy, full and fast-paced, that we rarely, if ever, become quiet or still enough to hear what our bodies want to tell us. In some cases, silence, rest or stillness are so uncomfortable, that we use the busy-ness, the constant noise and the social-media scrolling as a way to keep us distracted from ourselves and our over-thinking minds.

Over the past 15 plus years, I've studied, taught and shared a whole range of embodiment practices, I'm a trained well-woman therapist who has explored and who is forever exploring the body-mind psyche-spiritual connection, yet, despite knowing all I know, I *still* find myself disconnecting from my body and my experience as a woman.

This is how it usually goes for me.

I'll wake up, get out of bed, roll out my yoga mat, collect my phone from the office (I don't have tech in my room at night – see? My intentions are good!), but instead of pressing 'play' on a series of songs to support my morning practice of breath and movement (I know, so virtuous, right?), I open my emails instead.

I've barely opened my eyes and there's already a series of problems that I need to attend to. I go into reaction mode (fight or flight) and instantly I become overwhelmed. First about a specific thing (something that was mentioned in an email), but then, within a short amount of time, *everything* becomes overwhelming. (Our nervous system has a limited window in which it can tolerate intensity – good or bad – so because I'm not present, resourced in my body, the shock floods my system, creating overwhelm.)

So, I fire off a shitty, reactionary email (a defensive, ego-based reaction), sack off the morning practice entirely, put on the TV and drink a cup of coffee instead. I pretend I'm okay. I put on my 'I've got this' mask.

Except I haven't got this. Far from it.

The rest of the day gets messy (total freakin' understatement). That day turns into a week. Life gets dark. Really dark. All the coping mechanisms, rituals and techniques I've previously created in order to 'keep going and show up' fail.

I say really mean and hurtful things to myself about myself.

I get anxious, bitter and cynical about the world.

I eat. A lot. I numb out.

For many of us, the pattern I've described above, or at least a version of, is an everyday lived experience. You do what needs to be done in order to 'get by'. You react to and firefight problems. Your head, and its multitude of thoughts, think and overthink every situation and scenario to the point of exhaustion. You try to hold everything together so that you can keep your job and pay the bills; so that you appear successful and so that it looks as if your life is #squadgoals on social media (or for one of the gazillion other reasons you've been told that you need to keep going, producing, pushing and doing). Then you end up feeling really bloody inadequate, absolutely not good enough, stress your adrenals and you burn out because you simply can't keep it up.

Now, because of the work I do, I am able to realise when, how and why this happens. Sometimes it can take me an hour, sometimes it can take weeks, maybe even months, but thankfully, I do eventually realise. The point is it does still happen because that societal hypnosis? It's strong. Really strong, and it's why making time to connect with myself through breath and touch is now my first and non-negotiable daily act of both defiance and self-care. It's here that I can begin to slowly, and gently, start the process of stretching, nourishing and resourcing my nervous system and its capacity to tolerate more. That way, I'm able to come to every experience, every conversation, every interaction, (every potentially shitty email) feeling more grounded, more present to myself, to my body and her wisdom, which ultimately means I'm a less reactionary, less defensive human and there's potential for me to make smarter decisions and life choices. FYI: I say potential because I still mess up. I still make bad choices, but not as often. This is a practice. I repeat, this is a practice.

In a society that wants to keep us disconnected, moving, striving and doing, the idea of s–l–o–o–o–o–o–w–i–n–g down, resting – as in really resting, not scrolling on your phone or answering emails from your bed (yep, that's what I used to think resting was) –

BE.

HERE.

NOW.

IN YOUR BODY.
IN. THE. MOMENT.

is an act of boldness, because when you slow down, you're able to notice how you *feel*.

When you reconnect and actively engage with your body, its feelings and sensations, you're able to notice how you're feeling. In. The. Moment.

It's a practice that we can create for ourselves, with ourselves, that allows us to build the capacity to be present for more of our own experiences.

More joy.
More pleasure.
More love.
More sensuality.
More passion.
More creativity.

I invite you to take a pause right here and breathe.

———

NOTE: Many wellness and embodiment practices actively encourage you to take deep breaths and/or pay attention to your breathing. Now for most of us, slowing down and deepening the breath can be an instant self-soother, while for others, it can be really uncomfortable and create heightened anxiety in the body.

For instance, if you're feeling overwhelmed, a breath in for the count of four through your nose and a long, slow, drawn out exhalation for the count of eight can calm the nervous system. If you're feeling down and depressed, a more active breath may be more appropriate. If any kind of focused breathing is a problem for you, simply feel the air on your top lip as you breathe in and out at a pace that feels comfy for you.

INVITATION: S-L-O-W DOWN AND NOTICE

Take a look around you. Orientate yourself with the space you're in. Where's the door? What colours are the wall? Familiarising yourself with your surroundings creates a sense of safety. Keep your eyes open and, if it feels good to do so, breathe in through your nose and out through your nose. Let the tongue rest comfortably behind your teeth. Don't force anything. I like to place a hand on my heart and a hand on my womb space; the touch is soothing, supportive and reassuring.

———

What are you are noticing in your body? Is there anywhere that's tight? Sticky? Does anywhere feel soft?

Place a hand on your heart again and take a few more breaths.

Does anywhere feel hot or cold?

You don't have to do anything: you're simply noticing and honouring your current bodily state.

Try to give yourself a good five to ten minutes to notice all that needs to be noticed.

If it helps, you can try to name the sensations. *'Hmm, I feel a fizzy sensation to the left of my belly button.'* You could then, perhaps, sense if it has a colour. *'It's an orange-y colour.'*

I recommend doing this practice when you wake up (I do it while I'm still lying in bed – that way I can give myself NO excuses to get out of it). Then, if you can, create a few spaces in your day, even if it's for a minute or two, to take a few breaths and to check in with your body and its sensations.

This is a know-yourself-in-the-moment practice. The more you do it, the more familiar it becomes to observe, notice and name your state.

When you can name your state, you know yourself better. When you know yourself better, your body becomes a much safer place for you to inhabit.

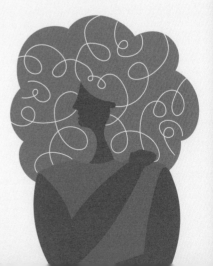

YOUR BODY AS A 'SAFE SPACE'

Safety comes from daily connectivity with yourself.

After the s-l-o-w down and notice practice, I add touch and movement. Nothing fancy, because if we make it too much of a 'thing', we don't do it, and what we *don't* want is for our morning connectivity practice to become another way in which we tell ourselves we're going to do something and then let ourselves down by *not* doing it. To create safety in the body we want super do-able micro rituals that encourage daily connectivity and trust. I tell myself 'I am loved and loveable' three times and put on a feel-good playlist, press 'shuffle' and stretch my body. Sometimes I sing along, sometimes I don't. Sometimes I shake – a good shake can really awaken your body. Sometimes I'll tap myself gently all over. Whatever I choose to do, I always move my body, specifically my hips, for at least three songs. And then? Well, then I sit still and quiet, letting myself be present and curious to all that is for five minutes. The sensations, the feels, the emotions.

What daily micro ritual could you do to create and build daily connectivity and trust with yourself?

When you feel safe in your body:

———— You move from hyper-aware 'reaction and survival' mode into a more relaxed 'rest and digest' mode. You breathe more deeply, your body feels less tight and constricted, and you can move freely and with ease.

———— You stop looking outside of yourself for answers and, instead, feel able to trust in your body's wisdom, rhythmic nature and guidance.

———— You are able to recognise the feelings of blame, shame, fear and humiliation (conditioning that can create such deep grooves in the psyches of so many women) dissipate and transmute when you dare to stay present. This way, it becomes possible to feel, to heal and accept *all* of your parts.

I AM
SAFE +
SUPPORTED

IN MY
BODY.

When you feel safe in your body, you can start to get curious.

You can ask your body questions and begin to listen to – and, more importantly, trust – its response. The insight you can receive helps you to gain vital intel on who you are and what it is you *really* need. Understanding how our bodies talk is how we can truly begin to grasp, honour and own our value and worth.

And that? Well, that's revolutionary.

BODY TALK

If you let it, your body's language can be a super smart, intuitive, inbuilt guidance system. (Which, in the face of so much uncertainty and chaos in the world right now, is really bloody needed.)

When you can tune in and listen to what your body has to say, and how she says it, you are able to soothe your nervous system, gently stretch it, move with it and expand its capacity for you to feel and experience more. What we're looking to do is to slowly (and with big love and compassion) connect with, and stay connected with, its sensations and its wisdom, so that if you ever find yourself feeling wobbly, fearful, confronted or challenged, or if you're experiencing uncertainty or not-knowing, you can self-regulate and find safety in your body.

LISTEN TO YOUR BODY. SHE KNOWS.

INVITATION: HUG AND HOLD

When we're held, we feel safe. So, I invite you to practise knowing that you can rely on yourself by regularly hugging and holding yourself.

———

Wrap your arms around yourself, crossing your arms against your chest. Breathe deep and long, and hold and squeeze yourself for as long as possible.

Say to yourself: 'I've got you.'

If you want some science-y stuff to back it up, giving yourself a big hug releases the happy hormones (oxytocin, serotonin and endorphins), which fill you up with good vibes. Honestly, though, it just feels bloody good – and we really should be doing more of the things that make us feel good, right?

ME TO MYSELF: I'VE GOT YOU

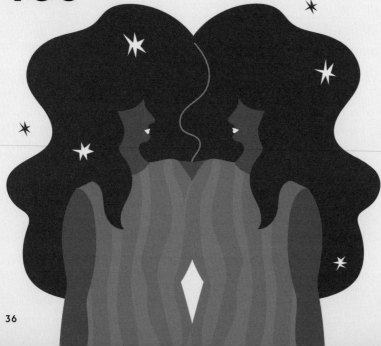

For many of us, when we disconnect from our bodies, we give our heads and the way that we think permission to run the entire life-living show. I don't know about you, but my ability to overthink is an extreme sport, and it's EXHAUSTING. Most of the decisions we make on a daily basis are automatic responses to what we've been taught throughout our lives: what's *supposedly* good or bad, right or wrong. These decisions are made by the part of the mind that's been conditioned by our life experiences, our thought systems and the beliefs that we have about the world we live in.

Your power is most potent when all your parts are present, online and witnessed. When the body and the mind work in collaboration and you have full access to your emotional, intuitive, spiritual and energetic pathways, this is you; powerful, present, whole and in your body.

It's here that you have the potential to make better choices. You can set strong boundaries. You're less likely to become overwhelmed when you experience challenges and difficult feelings. You can accept and honour what is, and you can creatively respond to life's challenges from a foundational place and space of safety.

YOU'RE POWERFUL, PRESENT AND WHOLE.

The work of choosing to stay present, connected and IN your body is a daily, lifelong practice of remembering. There isn't a one-size-fits-all, quick-fix process. We're humans, each with our own unique life experiences and sets of circumstances, so being present to how your body responds is powerful. This alone builds a relationship of trust with yourself. When you have trust in your body, you can stay present. When you stay present, you can start to experience yourself differently. Self-like – and even self-love – become possible. You can start to create a practice of reverence for the power of your own presence.

———

NOTE: If you're feeling some resistance and having thoughts like 'are you kidding me? I can't just trust my body all the time,' know that this is the habitual, binary, polarised, good-or-bad, right-or-wrong 'conditioned mind' talking. The truth is, at least in my experience, that when you let your body talk, and you make the decision to listen to your body at least some of the time, you gain access to a lot more information: inner-sourced wisdom, that is body-informed, based on your knowing and your intuition.

Basically, the really bloody good stuff.

2: FEEL THE FEELS
FEEL, REVEAL AND HEAL

Listening to – and trusting –
your body is a whole lot more
possible when you allow
yourself to fully experience
and express your wide-reaching,
ever-changing spectrum
of daily emotions.

How do you do that?

You dare to be present
to the feels.

THE FEAR OF FEELING

For many, the idea of *feeling our feelings* can create an instant full-body recoil. A question I am often asked is: 'What if it's too painful to feel?'

Honestly?

There's a chance it might be.

Most of us have, from an early age, been conditioned *not* to feel our emotions. We've also been taught that pain is *not* OK. We've been denied access to the feminine experience. (When I speak of the feminine, I speak of the deeply receptive feeling energy that's present in all of us, regardless of how you identify.) Yet that feminine experience contains the power of nature – the nature of our bodies, the nature of rhythm and cycles, the nature of the moon and the cosmos – and it's through this power that we can access all the deep and profound messages, codes and tools we need in order to be with, to make sense of and to process our emotions.

As a result of this conditioning, we have learned some really great and smart ways of *not* feeling.

Yep, more often than not, when the feels get *too* feely, we use some form of controlling behaviour to protect ourselves from the pain. The ways in which we do this come in many, many forms:

———— We stay in our heads rather than our bodies, because when we're in our heads we don't have to feel our feelings and we have a perceived, but unfortunately not always entirely accurate, sense of control.

———— We judge, shame or criticise ourselves to cover up what we're feeling.

———— We turn to various addictions – from substance use to addictive habits and behaviours – to numb out.

———— We hand our feelings over to someone else because we don't want to deal with them, or don't know how to.

Our work here – and yep, you've guessed it, it's the lifelong kind – is to unravel that conditioning, and reveal and welcome in, with BIG love, our emotions to be present and our feelings to be felt.

Exactly as they are.

How?

Well, there are a few ways – but my go-to method of choice
is to move.

MOVE TO FEEL

Your body is *meant* to move: it's primal, it's innate, it's necessary.

This is why I move my body every morning.
This is why I dance while doing the washing up.
This is why I shimmy my shoulders, shake my boobs and stamp
my feet whenever I hear a drum beat.

I teach and share yoga, somatic movement and *in-your-body-ment*
– my unique blend of nourishing movement designed specifically
to work in tune with the rhythmic intelligence of your body, but you
don't have to have any official training to move your body. It's what
your body is made to do! Women especially are wired to dance,
shake and move rhythmically – it's proven neuroscience – and when
we do, if we let it, dancing and moving our bodies is medicine.

My most favourite kind of movement happens when I make a
playlist – I consider playlists an art form and making them is one
of my personal superpowers – press play and let whatever feels
I'm feeling move with and through me. Basically, when you put
on music, you create potential space for your body to move and
f-e-e-e-e-l.

For example, if it's a super-upbeat playlist and I'm feeling pissed off,
I'll let the rhythm and sounds move my body. I'll let it create space
for me to feel into what's actually pissing me off. If I'm feeling rage,
anger, happiness, joy, overwhelm or any of the gazillion feels that
sit on the feeling spectrum, I move my body in ways that feel real,
supportive, nourishing and – most importantly – really bloody good.
I don't do this to get 'out' of my feelings, the act of movement
allows me to be revealed, for me to be with them and to most
importantly, f-e-e-l them.

LET IT BE MESSY.

THE EMOTIONAL REVEAL

Don't be afraid to let the process of feeling your feelings get messy: it *is* messy. And it's definitely *not* linear. Far, far from it.

Throughout *his*tory, we have been told that if we dare to feel or express our emotions – whether good or bad – we're 'crazy', 'over the top' and/or 'hysterical', so we've learned to numb them, push them down so that they don't 'spill over', so that we 'don't make a scene' or so that we're not seen as 'too much'.

It's why so many of us wear interchangeable masks: versions of ourselves that are deemed 'acceptable', made up of layer upon layer of thoughts, opinions and judgements from others about who we *should* be and how we *should* act.

It's also why so many of us, when asked to express ourselves, often don't know where to start. We've become so good at playing a role, of accepting the labels given to us by others, that we no longer recognise what's real. (Or, if we do, we're too afraid to be seen as who we really are, underneath all of *that*.)

So, yeah, it's definitely going to be messy – but consider the emotional reveal an opportunity to heal.

INVITATION: EXPLORE YOUR EMOTIONS

Use sound and movement to reveal and name your emotions. This process will support you in exploring the emotion that's revealed without going straight to your tried-and-tested programming.

———

Place a hand on your heart. Make sure the soles of your feet are firmly on the floor. If you're standing, bend slightly at the knees so that your knees aren't locked.

Breathe and be still.

Let any emotion, feeling or sensation make itself known to you and recognise where it is in your body. Is it in your tummy? Your left thigh? Your right elbow?

Can you name it? Is it disappointment? Resentment? Worry? Excitement?

Once you've done a full body scan of what's present, press shuffle on your favourite playlist.

Let whatever song that plays act as an oracle. Let the sounds and the words move into those places of the body where you'd noticed and named sensations. Allow your body to move and dance for the duration of the song. As you do so, listen to any messages you receive from your body.

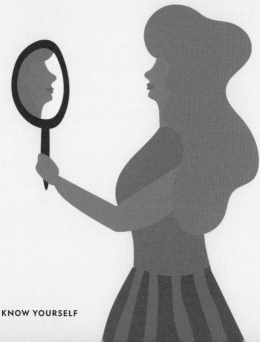

FEEL.
REVEAL.
HEAL.

I used to live a very fast-paced life. I worked long hours in TV and journalism while having to 'manage' (read: actively supress) my ever-present, oscillating feelings of 'I'm not good enough', imposter syndrome and constant, low-level anger and anxiety.

I found food to be quite useful at quietening the noise, saying yes made people like me (yep, recovering people-pleaser over here) and working long hours 'proved' that I was someone else's version of good enough.

This worked until... well, until it didn't.

Our bodies are always speaking to us, but if we continually ignore, stuff down and deny their cues, things can become toxic really quickly. And that pain we were/are trying so hard to avoid? Well, that can show up. Big time.

My avoidance and suppressed pain turned into what was, after many years of misdiagnosis, diagnosed as polycystic ovary syndrome (PCOS) and endometriosis. Yep, I'd stuffed my feelings of inadequacy, anger and not-good-enough so deep down that they showed up as physical pain and disease in my reproductive system. My story is not uncommon. In fact, many women that I work with as clients experience fertility and reproductive health issues – and 98 per cent of them are women who found themselves over-delivering in a male-dominated workplace in order to prove themselves 'good enough'.

I'm sharing this because it got gnarly.

It got gnarly because I was so busy trying to be a 'version' of myself that would be perceived as 'successful' and 'likeable' by the outside world, that I'd totally disconnected from my inner landscape – my body and my emotions – and I no longer had any idea as to who I actually was.

I was 26, and so I quit my job and went on an adventure. It was an adventure that has become life-long, exploring, navigating and healing my relationship with my body, power, pleasure and passion. I now support and guide other women as they make the same journey of self-exploration and discovery. For me, the PCOS and endometriosis was a massive kick in the vag and ovaries. My body's rather painful way of waking me up, getting me to pay attention, to remember who I was *before* I was told who I was.

It was my call home.

To my true nature.

Mother Nature.

RETURN TO NATURE – AND YOUR TRUE NATURE

Mumma Nature lets it *all* unfold.

She *knows*.

When we connect with the Great Mumma, we reconnect with source. Our own innate feminine power: the power to see, feel, hold and experience *all* that is; the power to know that we can handle the storm (and that, in some cases, we *are* the storm); and the power to know that *everything* has a season – a time to ebb, a time to flow, a time to be in action, a time to rest.

This is flow.

It's no wonder that we suffer and experience so much stress and toxicity in modern life. Our energies – physical, mental, emotional, spiritual and creative – have been forced into structures and systems that are masculine, goal-orientated and linear and simply don't allow for the natural flow of the feminine.

Yet when we turn to nature, when we observe nature, we remember.

The answer, whatever the question, is *always* nature.

She is source: she is the great, all-nourishing Mumma.

Connect with nature

Now, you don't need me to tell you how to do this – everyone has their own ways of creating a connection with nature – but here are some of *my* favourite ways to connect with the Great Mumma:

——— Go to the sea – salt water cures *everything*.

——— Listen to the birds sing – even in urban settings, you can hear birdsong. Yep, the squawk of a hungry seagull counts.

——— Plant herbs in the garden or on a windowsill – get your hands in the soil and plant rosemary and sage for starters. Then take cuttings, with love, to use in rituals, in baths and in your food.

——— Take baths. I am obsessed with baths. Intentional baths. Crystal, herbs and salt-infused baths. Daytime baths. Evening baths. ALL. THE. BATHS.

——— Follow the cycles and the phases of the moon – moon bathe and soak up her magic under the beams of the full moon, set intentions and co-create your visions for the future with her at the new moon.

Our cyclic nature

If you experience a menstrual cycle, it can be *the* most profound of ways to reconnect with your body and understand the rhythmic nature and flow of Mumma Nature as an emotional experience each month. That has been the case for me.

The menstrual cycle is *way* more than just a biological process; it's a cycle of ever-changing spiritual, emotional and creative energy. When you're present to the entire cycle (and not just the days that you bleed) you start to recognise that you experience life through the lens of the phase of the cycle that you're in at that moment in time: so how you see, feel and experience the world will change from week to week.

Yep, at each phase of your menstrual cycle, you show up to life differently. How I think and feel during my ovulation phase will be *very* different to how I think and feel during my menstruation phase. When you chart this, you can start to map patterns in what you feel and how you show up. This information can not only help you to manage and organise your life accordingly (total game changer); more importantly, it helps you to realise that, no, you're *not* consistent. In fact, you're consistently *not* consistent. And that's OK: consistency is an illusion. Oh, and guess what? You're not crazy, either. It's just that you've been boxed in and told to create, perform and act within restrictive, linear boundaries for far too long.

You're a woman, you're cyclic – and that is *not* a bad thing.

In fact, just so you know, it's a really bloody amazing thing. (Pun totally intended.)

I teach and share this wisdom in more depth and detail in my books *Code Red* and *Love Your Lady Landscape*, because cyclic intelligence is revelatory in helping us to remember that we have a built-in system that helps us to feel, reveal and heal our emotions each and every month. The good news is, you don't have to experience a menstrual cycle to connect with the cyclic nature of, well, nature, because the menstrual cycle is mirrored in the phases of womanhood, the cycles of the moon and the seasons of Mumma Nature. We can work with any – or all – of them to return to our true nature and explore our feelings.

INVITATION: SHE-SCAPE

You have cyclic intelligence available to you that will help you to make sense of WTF is going on and what you're feeling in any given moment, both personally and collectively. Every day, you can track what I call your 'she-scape' – the daily landscape of *you*. It becomes a personalised and, more importantly, a felt-in-your-body forecast for the day ahead.

———

To explore your she-scape, take a breath, place a hand on your heart and ask yourself the following questions:

• How are you feeling?

• Where are you feeling it?

• If you experience a menstrual cycle, what day of the cycle are you on? (Tracking your cycle helps you to know what phase you're in, and it may help you to understand why you're feeling a particular way. For example, when I'm on day 25, I'm premenstrual and often full of rage. If you keep track of your cycle for a few months, you'll start to see patterns emerge. (For more information on tracking and what each

phase means, go to my website: www.thesassyshe.com.)

• What phase is the moon in?

• What astrological sign is the moon in? (You can use apps like iLuna that will send you a notification when the moon changes phase, as well as what astrological sign it is in – this changes every 2½ days and can have a major impact on our moods and emotions.)[2]

• What season is it?

Use the table on the next page to see the links between the way you're feeling and the seasons, moon phases and your own menstrual cycle. Tracking your cyclic intel in this way can help you to build a relationship of trust with your inner landscape. It can help you to make sense of your current experience, in the moment; to realise that it's ever-changing, which will hopefully help you to understand yourself better and to be a little easier on yourself in the process.

[2] You can, if you wish, turn your direction to the wider cosmos and check planet placement, too. I'm an astro-geek, so in my online community, the SHE Power Collective, I share how what's going on 'up there' influences things 'down here'. If you want to explore for yourself, you can use a phone app like Time Passages or Astro Gold.

Season	SPRING	SUMMER	AUTUMN/FALL	WINTER
Womanhood phases	Maiden Minx – curious and sensual	Mumma Creatrix – fertile and fecund	Wise Wild – untamed and without a filter	Crone All-knowing – cares very little for societal expectations
Moon phases	Waxing	Full	Waning	Dark
Menstrual cycle phases	Pre-ovulation	Ovulation	Pre-menstruation	Menstruation
Action	Growth – plant new seeds and tend to them Curiosity – open to new experiences and willing to try new things	Creation and manifestation – turning dreams and ideas into reality	Revealing – seeing everything exactly as it is Shedding – letting go	Death and rebirth – surrender and new beginnings Dream time – visioning
Feelings	Optimistic Daring Like anything is possible	Self-assured Positive Confident	Sharp tongue No bullshit Discerning Bad bitch	Soft Dreamy Contemplative

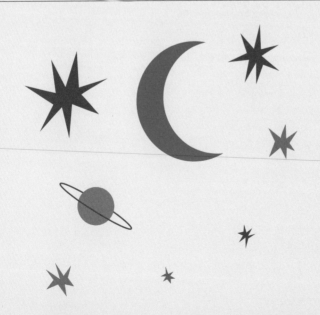

GET COMFORTABLE WITH THE UNCOMFORTABLE

Yes, feeling your feelings *might* – ha! Who am I trying to kid? – *will* mean having to get comfortable with the uncomfortable, but understanding that the pain *won't* actually consume you (no matter how much you think it might) will help you to become present to your current experience. At the same time, it's important to remember that your feelings and current experience can – and undoubtedly will – be subject to change in any given moment, and you have to get comfortable with that, too.

Your feelings get bigger when you:

———— resist them
———— avoid them
———— judge them
———— ignore them
———— criticise them
———— deny them

Your feelings are more 'feel'-able when you:

———— get curious about them
———— allow them to be present
———— meet them where they are in your body
———— acknowledge and name them

When we feel the feelings, we learn that we can tolerate them, even the hard ones. This allows us to build up an inner strength, resolve and resilience as the feeling moves through us, rather than stay stuck inside of us.

Obviously, this too takes practice; it's all practice, that's the point. Take it slow, start over as many times as you need to, and don't believe you have to feel it (whatever 'it' is) alone. You *can* ask for help and support – in fact, I actively encourage it. A trained therapist/coach/somatic practitioner can support, guide and help you to create a safe space for you to experience and feel your feelings.

———

NOTE: I know that I've only talked about the painful and gnarly feels so far, and that's because they're usually the ones that get pushed down and ignored and turn toxic. But I'm also aware that, for many of us, feeling the good feels – joy, happiness, possibility – can be tricky too. Don't worry: I've got you. We're going to be exploring the good feels when we source ourselves in chapter 5.

3: FLIP THE SCRIPT
RETELLING YOUR STORY

Every day, in every moment, the many, many stories we've been told about ourselves – and believe to be true – are playing on a repeating loop in our minds. These are stories that are made up of the beliefs, expectations and projections of others; stories passed down through our family lineage; stories that we've been told or that we've borrowed from the place where we grew up, or have been heavily suggested to us through our culture and the society we live in.

This is what Professor Jerome Bruner, a Harvard psychologist, terms 'narrative discourse'. A process by which we construct our values and beliefs from the external input that we receive. Basically, our brains are designed to learn from stories. They tell us who we are and how we fit within our family, our friendship groups, our culture and the collective. We take these stories, and we live them out. With each lived out moment, they are retold and become deeply embedded, as if they're factually correct. This unfortunately leaves very little room for you to control your narrative as the unique and special human that you are.

The thing is, when you listen to your body wisdom, when you're aligned to your real-to-you frequency, you will know, deep, deep down in your belly, at your centre, in the place where you connect to your truest nature, when the stories that you've been led to believe are not your truth, because you f-e-e-e-l it.

But remember that societal hypnotism I spoke about earlier? It has us all under its spell. Author, branding expert and cultural commentator Seth Godin speaks to this 'spell' in his altMBA seminar, 'People like us (do things like this) Change a culture, change your world'. He suggests that the things that you are told that people like *you* do become woven into the fabric of your stories. They gain strength and momentum there, and it's there that they become fact.

INVITATION:
WHAT'S YOUR STORY?

What is your current
story about:

- money?
- family?
- relationships?
- your body?
- your health?
- work?

—

Take a paper and pen and set
a timer for 15 minutes. Ask
yourself: *What is my current
story about money?* And then
write the first thing that comes
up for you. Keep going, working
your way through the list. No
judgement: don't get too caught
up in the details. Simply allow
a few minutes for each story
to unfold.

*To make money you have
to work really hard.*

*To be loveable you have
to be thin, popular and beautiful.*

*To be spiritual you have
to speak in a breath-y yoga
teacher voice, wear tie-dye
and chant every morning
at 4 a.m. to a designated deity.*

These are just some of the
stories I was told and believed
to be true for the longest time:
but what I know now is that
my life, and my experience
of it, is dependent on the
story that *I* choose to tell.

What you think and speak
creates your reality, so I take
radical responsibility, on a daily
basis, to monitor my thoughts,
get really intentional and speak
the life I want to live – a life lived
in total alignment with who I am
– into existence.

A life that resonates
at *my* frequency.

Because *I* get to choose.

The good news?
You get to choose, too.

YOU GET TO CHOOSE THE STORY YOU TELL.

AND THE LIFE THAT YOU LIVE.

If your current stories feel deeply uncomfortable and out of alignment with your truth and your big, beautiful heart and belly-deep wisdom, yet you find that you're playing them over and over on repeat in your life (and in your body), you get to flip the script and tell a different story.

You get to choose what you believe to be true about yourself, the life you live and the way you choose to live it.

DROP THE 'SHOULDS'

When you follow the 'shoulds' – I 'should' weigh ten pounds less, I 'should' have x number of social media followers – you censor your inner desires and you disconnect from your body and your true-to-you wants and needs. If you've ever found yourself saying 'I don't know what I want', it's because you're following the 'shoulds' and *not* your own inner wisdom.

This isn't your fault. We're told that the 'shoulds' are the 'right' and 'safe' thing to do, and for a while, we play along. Yet, as you reconnect to your body and you feel your feelings, you'll find that those things you've been told you 'should' be doing can become really uncomfortable – because they're *not yours*.

If we could drop the 'shoulds', we would destroy the script of everything we've been told and sold as women. Let's imagine *that* for a hot minute.

It can be hard at first to identify the 'shoulds', because they often pretend that they actually *are* your needs and wants – I know, sneaky, right? They usually, although not exclusively, show up when you're doubting yourself or feeling silenced or uncomfy in your body. Identifying your 'shoulds' is *not* a one-time task: it's about recognising the current stories that you're telling yourself and seeing where the 'shoulds' are showing up within them. This is why being *in* your body and trusting its wisdom is so important: because, if you let it, your body really can *feel* when something doesn't align with who you are and what it wants.

JUDGEMENT AND COMPARISON

When you're living someone else's story, your life becomes a really hard, *not* fun and definitely *not* juicy experience. Actual fact.

Yet, I defy anyone to tell me that they haven't, at one point or another, found themselves comparing their own lives and stories to those of others, especially on social media, and judging themselves accordingly.

How can we not? The whole system is set up to keep us scrolling, to make us want things we don't need, and to make us think things we didn't even know we thought.

I won't go into the science and psychology of social media – it's a total 'thing' – but when our lived experience and the stories that we're telling don't match up with our truth, our frequency and our body wisdom, it's time to consider the impact that social media is having. These platforms are definitely where many of us find ourselves in a state of blame, shame, judgement and comparison: both of ourselves and of each other.

Here's the deal. Our social nervous system is the part of the body's control centre that allows us to read and respond to our environment. In order for this social nervous system to be at ease, we need to know who we are in relation to everyone around us. We want to feel safe, like we belong, and that people understand us and accept us. When we question that, or someone says something to make us feel like we don't belong and aren't accepted, we get stuck in judgement and comparison states.

FYI: This is a super-simplified version of Dr Stephen Porges' very complex and incredibly powerful Polyvagal Theory. If you want to geek out on what's essentially the science of feeling safe, two of my favourite teachers and humans, Deb Dana and Amber Gray, both do incredible work in this field, too.

Your social nervous system is ruled from the heart up – neck, throat, jaw, ears and eyes – and it's here that you may notice feelings and sensations of judgement and comparison show up, so pay attention.

If ever you notice yourself getting judge-y, or comparing yourself to someone else, place a hand on your heart and tell yourself, 'I am safe in my body, I belong here.' Do this three times.

When you feel safe, you're able to make space for compassion.

When there's compassion, we no longer feel so threatened, so we're able to move out of judgement and comparison. Essentially, we become a whole lot less critical of both ourselves and others, and instead make space to become a whole lot more empathetic and understanding.

The truth? We're all doing the best we can. Our lives, and the way we live them, are all affected by stories, our childhoods, trauma, and past events and experiences. What we experience of someone in person, or what they share on social media, is only what they have chosen to share in that moment. We are forever changing, from moment to moment. We learn new things, we do better, we mess up, we make different choices, we experience new people and places – and guess what? We change our minds.

There is never simply one version of who we are. Each of us is multi-layered, beautiful, messy, complex and ever-evolving. And thank bloody goodness for that.

WE'RE ALL DOING THE BEST WE CAN.

LET'S ALL CUT OURSELVES A LITTLE SLACK, YEAH?

YOU MAKE THE RULES

I personally live by these words shared by the incredibly talented English actor, Helen McCrory: 'How should a woman live her life? Survive to the age of 70, fearfully, being as everyone else instructs her to be? Or play the heroine, passionately, in the knowledge that trying and failing need not equal defeat?'

You do not have to sign up to a prescribed set of rules and instructions about what you should do and who you should be. You get to write, and most importantly, live by your own set of rules.

Here's mine:

———— I drink gin *and* I do yoga.

———— I meditate each morning *and* I watch *Real Housewives* (the entire franchise – every season, every locale).

———— I'm fat *and* I'm fit.

———— I have a big heart *and* I have fierce boundaries.

———— I love hot pink acrylic nails *and* I do moon rituals.

———— I study Jung *and* I read romantic fiction.

We don't have to be this *or* that – we can be this *and* that.

We can be all our parts, without any justification. How good does *that* feel?

Now, with that in mind, what story will *you* tell?

RETELLING YOUR STORY

Yep, the story you tell is up to you.

You have the capacity to speak and create your reality into being. Now, this can be tricky, because oftentimes, so much of who we believe we are is caught up in the old stories and narratives. Also, and this might be really ouch-y to hear, these stories and narratives can support and justify behaviours that we might have become really quite attached to – so be gentle with yourself as you explore and allow yourself to get curious about retelling your story.

Because my family was poor and I grew up on a council estate, a story I used to tell was that making money was hard. By telling that story, the pay-off for me was that I was always right. Because it is hard to make money when that's the story I tell over and over again.

When I took away my need to be right, when I recognised that my parents' story didn't have to be *my* story, when I chose to repeat 'making money is easy for me' three times before I went to bed each night (whether I believed it or not – and at first I definitely didn't!), I created space for a different outcome.

By re-writing your narrative, you're not deleting all the things that you've done or have been, you are simply opening yourself up to what's possible while taking fierce self-responsibility for what comes next. You are fully accepting your role as a creatrix, a manifesting maven, one who is collaborating with her heart and belly wisdom, source and the cosmos to create a different possibility.

––––––

When you tell your story the way *you* want it to go,
you take back your power.

When someone tries to give you a label but you
refuse to accept it as truth,
you take back your power.

When you set clear intentions about what and who you
let into your life, what feels good and what serves you,
you take back your power.

It doesn't mean that bad things won't and don't happen, or that events like a global pandemic won't come along and completely side-swipe all your best laid plans while bringing up a ton of trauma that you thought you'd previously resolved. They will – you're a human, having a human experience. But your power, your *presence*, is held in the story *you* choose tell.

––––––

NOTE: I am not saying you can simply think a positive thought, say a positive affirmation, click your fingers and positive things will 'magically' happen and manifest. This is about recognising that, in the process of de-programming the societal spell (and that's definitely not going to happen overnight), whatever story you choose to believe about yourself and play on repeat will always be your truth.

'I don't deserve to be successful' and 'I deserve to be successful' both have the potential to be true stories – which one will you choose to play on repeat?

YOU HAVE PERMISSION TO CHOOSE A DIFFERENT STORY.

(YOU DON'T *NEED* PERMISSION,
BUT JUST IN CASE YOU'RE SEEKING IT, HERE IT IS.)

INVITATION:
TELL YOUR STORY,
CLAIM YOUR POWER

Set aside some time for yourself, with a journal and pen, and feeling safe and like you belong in your own body, without judgement or comparison, give yourself a full body shake, hydrate, gently tap your heart three times with the palm of your hand and drop into stillness.

Ask yourself the following question: 'Body, from this place of vital creation, possibility and opportunity, what's the story I now want to tell about':

- money?
- family?
- relationships?
- my body?
- my health?
- work?

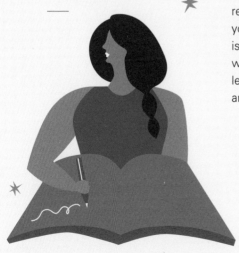

Then, writing in the present tense, using words from your own vocabulary and writing events, situations and scenarios as if they are already true, be clear, intentional and really descriptive about how you actually want your life to be: when you're not doing it for 'likes' and followers on social media; when you're not doing it to meet parental or familial expectations; when you're doing it your way, on your own terms.

Tell the story of successful, satiated, soul-nourished *you*.

It might be that this particular story isn't too far from your current reality, or it may feel like they're a gazillion miles apart. Either way, read your story to yourself daily – when you wake up, and when you go to bed, when you're waiting in the bus queue, when you're having a tea break – because the story you repeat over and over, the story you breathe life and vitality into, is the story that your frequency will respond to and meet. So, let's make it as juicy, nourishing and vital as possible, yeah?!

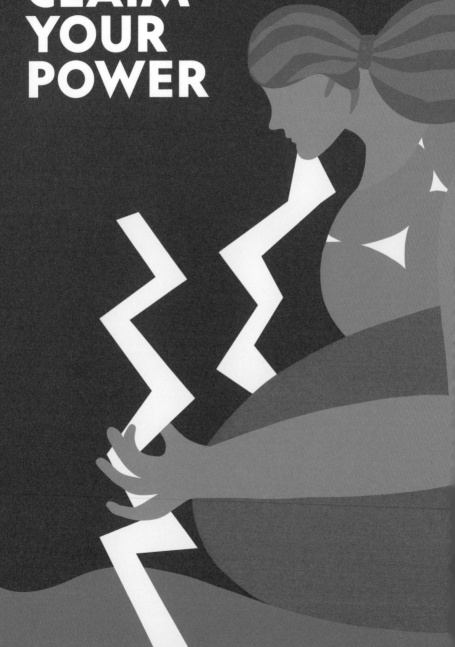

PART TWO:
CLAIM
YOUR
POWER

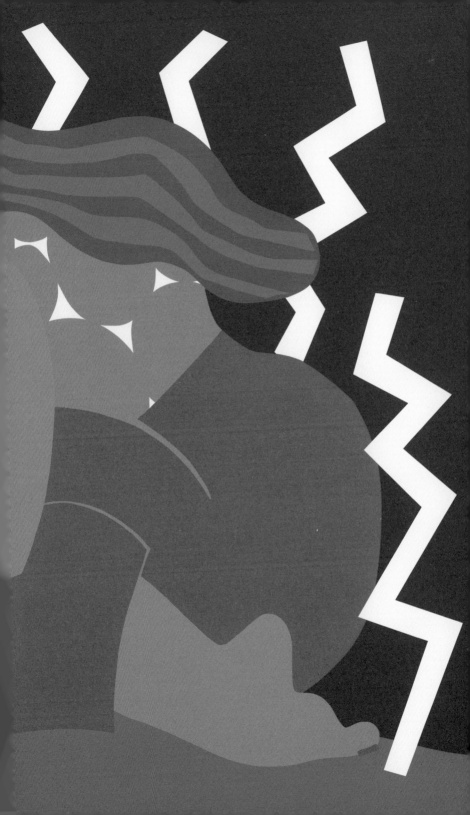

4: FIND YOUR FREQUENCY

Connect to your
centre and locate
your own,
unique-to-you
energy source

In the spiritual and wellness worlds, you will often hear the terms 'high-vibe' and 'raise your vibrations' or 'good vibes only'. The idea being that you somehow need to be elevated from a perceived 'lower vibration' or state of being.

The truth is, you are *always* vibe-ing.

YOU ARE A VIBE.

Ru Paul says: '*Honey, you're an energetic phenomenon.*'
Yep, you are, quite literally, a vibe. As your heart beats, it sends out a vibration, a drumbeat, through your entire body, over and over and over again. It's a resonation of your true-to-you frequency.

So, instead of needing to vibrate 'higher' or 'better' by drinking a green juice, holding a yoga pose for 20 minutes or eating an 'activated' food item of some description, what if you tuned into your heart, located your true centre, distinguished *your* vibration and rhythmic intelligence, and resonated, received, transmitted, created, magnetised, shared and lived fully at *your* frequency?

THE BEAT OF
YOUR HEART

+

THE TRUTH OF
YOUR BELLY

=

YOUR
FREQUENCY.

WHAT'S YOUR FREQUENCY?

I believe your frequency is your total you-ness in energetic, vibratory form. The stronger the vibration, the stronger your frequency.

It's when the beat of your heart aligns with the truth of your belly. It affects your posture, your breath, how you receive, your sensorial awareness, how you orgasm, how you listen, how you think and how you communicate with the world. It's who you are at your very core, when all the false programming has been released, layers of facades and stories have been unfurled and the tension, the anxiety, the guilt and the need to please has been dropped. It's the source of your passion, creativity, courage, confidence and capacity to love – and it activates your intuition, insight and sense of purpose. It's your connection to the source of life itself. Therefore, it's your source of power. Your power force. (I mean, no big deal, right?)

The quieter you become, the more you can hear.

NOTE: Both Ram Dass and Rumi are credited with this quote: I love both equally and feel like they'd have both said it, so choose your own favourite whisperer of wise words.

FEELING CENTRED

The information overload we experience on a daily basis is real.
Unless we find a way to make some space for stillness and quiet
in our lives, it can become very difficult, very quickly, to figure out
what actually belongs to us and what is just being pushed on to
us. Is that my thought? Is that my reality? So the act of tuning in,
whether it's for ten minutes with your hand on your heart in silence,
placing your bare feet on the grass, or a two-hour breath and
meditation session, can help you to become present at your centre.

When you're centred, there's no resistance. You're present to what
is. You can breathe more deeply. You have more capacity to expand
and grow. You feel stronger. You're alive and alert, and you're able
to fully align with, and tune into, your frequency.

You know you're not centred if you:

——— react and lash out without thinking;
——— scroll on your phone *all the time*;
——— feel overwhelmed by everything;
——— are easily distracted and find you just can't focus;
——— look to others to solve your problems; and
——— speak negatively about yourself, to yourself.

When we're not centred, it's much harder to trust ourselves.
We disconnect from our instincts and our inner knowing, and
we don't respond well to the inevitable ups and downs of life.
This forces us to either future-trip – in other words, to endlessly
worry and try to control what 'might' happen in the future –
or to ruminate and dwell on what's happened in the past.
Both of which, FYI, we have absolutely no control over.

When we're centred, though, we can turn down the outside
'noise' and tune in to our own frequency. We're embodied.
We're anchored. We're present. And it's here that we become
our own sacred ground.

BE YOUR OWN SACRED GROUND.

LOCATE YOUR CENTRE

Your physical centre is located at the core of your being, in your belly. Societal rules have dictated that women should hold their bellies in, should aim to cultivate a tight, washboard-like stomach, and should feel some kind of self-loathing towards their bellies – but we're dropping those 'shoulds', remember? Back in the day, a beautiful round belly and the power held within it was admired and revered. In Greek mythology, the goddess Baubo – who is basically a glorious belly on legs with nipples for eyes and a vulva for a mouth – bares her belly, tells dirty jokes, wiggles her hips and lifts her skirt to flash her vulva (my kind of goddess!). The belly laughter that she evokes by doing this means that the life force and fecundity of the land (along with the life force and fecundity in the bellies of all women) are restored and thrive. Hurrah!

INVITATION: CONNECT WITH YOUR BELLY

To reclaim your belly as your instinctual voice of knowing and wisdom, locate your centre and start to connect with – and trust – your gut.

———

Breathe naturally and bring a hand, or both hands, palms down, to the space approximately 5 cm (2 inches) below your belly button.

Bring your awareness to the space beneath your palms and take slow, rhythmic breaths from your belly. If you rarely connect with this part of your body, this might create tension. If so, begin by breathing from your chest a few times first, then focus on moving down to your belly.

Keep taking these slow, rhythmic belly breaths for between three and five minutes.

Depending on your current relationship with your tummy, this exercise can activate stuck feelings and emotions. Don't be afraid: let them surface, witness them and be gentle with yourself in the process. Reclaiming your relationship with your beautiful belly as your wisdom centre is a process – remember that.

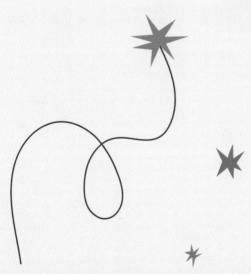

TRUST YOUR INTUITION

Your intuition is a 'gut instinct', felt at your centre. Your belly has its own nervous system – the enteric nervous system, ENS – and it's here that we feel 'butterflies' when we're excited or experience the 'drop of dread' sensation when we receive bad news. I like to think of it as our '*inner*-tuition': an internal guidance system that's always teaching us and providing us with deeper insight and understanding about what's going on in our lives. It knows exactly what you really want. It can give you the heads-up on possible opportunities that feel good and aligned, and it can sound the sirens if something is a definite no-go. Lots of people hear it like an inner voice, others experience it as bodily feelings and sensations. And many of us ignore it and shut it down, because we've been told that rational thinking is the 'right' way to think.

How do you know the difference between gut instinct and rational thought? You let your body tell you.

If you're all up in your head, overthinking and fear-filled, you may feel frustration, confusion and possible anxiety. If you're down in your gut, you probably won't be able to make sense of what you're feeling with rational thought, but it will feel instantly 'right' and 'true'.

Learning to recognise what your own intuition feels or sounds like... wait for it... takes practice.

If I'm seeking guidance, I'll place my hands below my navel, breathe deeply and hum. Why? Because when you hum, or meditatively 'om', your voice box vibrates, sending out a 'relax and chill' signal to the nervous system. As your body relaxes, it becomes easier for you to access the wisdom of your belly (versus the noise in your head).

I then ask my belly and her deep knowing for guidance.

Sometimes I'll hear a word or a phrase or even a fully formed sentence, but if I'm honest, that doesn't happen nearly as often as I'd like. Most of the time, I experience it as sensations rather than words. If something is not okay, I'll get a sharp, sinking feeling at the pit of my tummy; if it's positive, I'll get warm tingling sensations from hip to hip; and if it needs more thought, I'll feel an urge to rub my belly in a nurturing way. If, for some reason, nothing comes through, I recognise that there's a really big chance I don't want to hear the answer, so, and this is something I learnt from one of my most favourite humans, Shaman Durek, I say out loud: 'I release any fear of hearing the answer' and then I ask the question out loud again. It may take a few goes, but it works!

I AM CENTRED, ALIGNED AND SELF-ASSURED.

THE HEART AND GUTS OF YOU

Your frequency will be different to the frequencies of others. *That's* the idea.

When you tune into and resonate at your specific, true-to-you frequency, it means you might not say or do the same things as other people. Your thoughts and opinions might be different; and the actions you choose to take, or not take, might not be the same, either.

Good.

What happens when you're connected at your heart and centred in your belly is that your inner guidance is amplified and you become aligned with your frequency. Your posture changes, you stand taller, you breathe more deeply, you feel confident and self-assured, and what you speak in the world has a strong, clear, real, uplifting and true-to-you resonance.

You trust it.

Others trust it, too.

This is *you*, centred and aligned. How good does that feel?

When you vibrate at your own frequency:

—— you're present, and that presence becomes powerful;

—— it's much harder to manipulate you (even though people may still try);

—— you can hold more of the whole human experience (and recognise that it's messy, that it's not as simple as this *or* that – there are multitudes of realities and possibilities);

—— it's easier for you to recognise what you're willing to accept as your responsibility (and what you're definitely not willing to allow be projected upon you);

—— you stay centred and in your body for longer (and it feels good, not uncomfortable); and

—— it's harder to knock you – criticism has a little less impact.

REAL TALK: HATERS GONNA HATE

When you do vibrate at your own frequency, criticism and negative feedback (that's my polite way of saying haters) *will* have a little less impact on you – but they will still undoubtedly happen. In fact – real talk – there's a chance you could experience them more.

It's why so many of us hide or shy away from being present and sharing our powerful presence in the world. After all, those stories we have been conditioned to tell ourselves, and the many masks we have been taught to wear – they all keep us safe, right?

No one wants to actively put themselves out there if there's even the slightest possibility of not being liked, getting attacked or hated on, do they? Yet, that fear of being noticed, seen or criticised, just for doing/believing/being something/someone different is what keeps so many of us from truly expressing ourselves and living our most full, juicy and joyful lives.

WHAT PEOPLE THINK OF YOU IS NOT YOUR PROBLEM –

OR YOUR RESPONSIBILITY.

THE WORLD NEEDS YOU TO RESONATE AT YOUR FREQUENCY.

As someone who has written books, shared her art in the world and stood on a stage in front of hundreds of people, yes, I can wholeheartedly confirm that criticism, rejection and hate hurt. A lot. And… I can also confirm that, when I'm aligned and centred and vibrating at my frequency, they definitely hurt a lot less – because I know and trust myself.

Haters will *always* hate. Especially if your frequency transmission vibrates differently to theirs.

Of course, sometimes people simply don't like you, or, because of their own 'stuff', they misunderstand you, or they don't agree and are not open to seeing what's being said or shared from any perspective apart from their own. But, for the most part, it's because by vibrating at your own frequency and transmitting that to the world, you will highlight what they're *not* doing and being in the world and what they may or may not be willing and/or ready to take responsibility for yet or ever.

But there is good news. Yes, there is *definitely* good news. You will also become a beacon of mother-loving light. Like-attracts-like. Those who vibrate and resonate with all that you are and share in the world will want to know you, learn from you, spend time with you and lift you up. Yep, the more strongly you vibrate and resonate at your own frequency, the more magnetic and powerful your presence will become.

You literally cannot help it.

5: SOURCE YOURSELF

Resource,
nourish
and nurture

In the past, I have been what's commonly referred to as a 'self-help' obsessive. All the formulas, all the protocols, all the many, many ways to make myself 'better' (most of which usually involved me buying products, or paying for a course or training of some description). You name it, I've done it. I've drunk the juices; I've bought the books; I've done the online programmes; I've put the very, very expensive cream on my face; I've bought the pillows that promise better sleep; I've gone to workshops up mountains; I've danced naked; I've worn the crystals (not going to lie, I'm never *not* going to wear the crystals). And, while some of the above have definitely made me feel better (for a while, at least), rarely has any of it left me feeling fully satiated, deep in my belly – my centre – for long periods of time. So, I'd continue my search for the next self-help-wellness dopamine and serotonin hit, the next miracle product or teacher, the next thing that was going to give me a temporary sense of feeling-better-ness (while ultimately leading to me berating myself for not being able to keep up with and maintain the programme/the green juice regime/the five-point plan).

Rinse and repeat, rinse and repeat, rinse and repeat.

And I *know* I am not alone.

Self-help, which has now basically been rebranded as self-care, has become a gazillion-dollar industry that is less about your *actual* needs and well-being and much more about making the dollar-dollar by encouraging you – with the help of influencers and pretty images on social media – to buy 'stuff' for your *perceived* needs and well-being.

Now, I'm not for one minute suggesting that self-care isn't important. It is. Self-care is *really* bloody important. Essential, in fact. But in order for it to be supportive and nourishing and replenishing, it has to be self-care on *your* terms, not a five-step formula or a one-size-fits-all protocol put together by someone who doesn't even know you and doesn't take into account your specific needs, wants and requirements.

CONNECT TO SOURCE

Self-sourcing, a term I coined in my book, *Witch*, is my response to the bombardment of all the ways in which we are told to help, care for and love ourselves.

By the way, I'm not saying that you *don't* do any of the things we've been told make us feel better: I love taking baths, I ritualise the shit out of everything, I *still* buy expensive beauty products and perfume and often take retreats in the middle of bloody nowhere. What I *am* saying is that when we understand when, and how, we're being sold to, that we get to know ourselves well enough that we can be responsive. We can align with source, practise discernment and trust ourselves to make informed, from-the-gut, fully embodied decisions about what nourishment we *actually* need and want.

What I know about myself is that:

———— a 20-minute dance-off with myself is as beneficial, if not more so, than me doing Pilates simply because I've been told that Pilates is good for me.

———— 10 minutes of sun-soaked stillness in my garden with the soles of my feet in the dirt of Mumma Earth is as beneficial, if not more so, than holding a yoga pose for the same amount of time.

———— making art with felt-tip pens is as potent, if not more so, than a deep, eyes shut, hour-long meditation.

———— drinking a cup of ceremonial cacao with coconut cream and a dash of rosewater, slowly and intentionally, is as beneficial, if not more so, than a calorie/fat/all-the-things-controlled eating regime. (And, just so you know, cacao contains more calcium than cows' milk, is packed with iron, magnesium and antioxidants, and can help with issues such as depression, stress, blood pressure and heart health. I LOVE cacao. Can you tell?)

This is *my* truth. You might find that Pilates and an hour-long meditation is the most incredible way to show your body love, which is why connecting to source – through your intuitive belly knowing – and resourcing yourself from there is an individual, gut-led, trust-the-body assessment of what nourishes *you* specifically.

Self-sourcing involves a deep honouring of your physical, emotional, psychological and spiritual state, in any given moment, and tending to it accordingly.

Gather data on yourself.

Tracking your she-scape daily, as we explored on page 51, can really help you to witness where there are patterns and rhythms that you can respond to. Our cyclic and rhythmic nature and intelligence mean that our needs and wants can actually become somewhat predictable. Knowing this helps us to resource ourselves accordingly. When I'm on day one of my menstrual cycle, for example, heat pads, cacao, rest and lots of silence make me feel good and nourished. When I get anxious and start feeling out of control, I take a salt bath, slow my breath and probably cry. A lot. When I want to manifest something important in my life, I bring myself to orgasm. When I'm feeling down and unmotivated, I put on Lizzo's 'Good as Hell' and tell myself, 'Three minutes; just move your body for three minutes.' It's a state-shifter.

We're living in interesting/uncertain/somewhat wild times, and the more we know how to source our own nourishment – whether that's through giving ourselves a hug when we get overwhelmed by what we hear on the news, dancing and stamping out feelings of rage, or growing our own fruit and veg (I cannot tell you how much joy and nourishment I've received from tending to, singing to and then actually being able to eat my own tomatoes, raspberries, strawberries, broccoli and garlic) – the more we are able to stay steady, centred and sourced.

It's a lifelong, ever-changing exploration of what brings you joy, what lights you up, what nourishes you, what makes you feel really good – and it's your self-written permission slip to go get them.

COME TO YOUR SENSES

Sometimes I can smell someone's body odour from three metres away. Sometimes I can hear every single conversation in a restaurant. Sometimes my skin comes out in hives simply by my being in proximity to something or someone I don't like. Some call this heightened sensitivity; some call it a spiritual superpower. But honestly? I used to think it meant I was bloody crazy.

It turns out, though, that people who experience hypermobility – that's me, I'm hypermobile – also have a tendency to experience a hyper-alert sensorial nature, too.

Wild, huh?

You don't need to be hypermobile to become sensorially alert. But for me, my experience of having a hyper-alert sensorial nature has highlighted the power of our senses and how vital they are to the flavour and quality of our frequency and presence.

I have all my best ideas in the shower, when warm water is kissing my skin. Diffusing essential oils like frankincense and myrrh helps to clear my mind and evoke clarity. Seeing my books organised by colour on their shelves puts me at ease. The smell of jasmine and ylang ylang makes me feel all kinds of sexy. Seeing roses in my garden makes me feel loved. Wearing hot pink accessories feels powerful *and* fun. Tasting cacao soothes my heart. We can all use sounds, feelings, sights, tastes and smells to connect with our bodies, to reveal and heal our emotions and to make decisions about what it is we really need, want and desire.

INVITATION: PRESENT SENSE

If you've ever had therapy, there's a good chance your therapist shared this exercise with you. Mine did, and it's a really simple and effective way to tune into your senses and to recognise which of your senses are your strongest. (FYI: There are five traditional senses – touch, sight, hearing, smell and taste – but according to scientists doing important research, there's potentially more than 20 senses for us to explore!)

——

Find a quiet place to sit.

Take in some big deep breaths and place your hands on your belly. Let it be soft as you breathe in and breathe out.

Look around you. Find five things that catch your eye, and name them.

Next, notice four sensations you're currently feeling in your body, and name them.

Now, find three sounds that you can hear, and name them.

Identify two emotions that you're currently experiencing, and name them.

Finally, find one thing you can taste in your mouth, and name it.

This practice brings you into your body and the 'felt' sense of your current experience. In doing so, it brings you into the present moment so you can be... well, present.

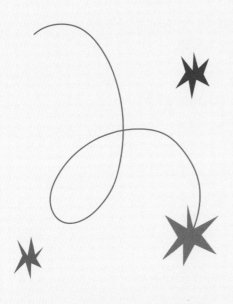

Sensorial pleasure

Now that you're present and your senses are alert, make a list of the things that heighten *your* senses and that *your* body responds to positively.

It can be a smell – I am obsessed with the scent of rose and oud. It might be the act of putting on moisturiser after a shower and whispering 'I love you' to each body part as you do it. It might be walking through a bluebell-filled wood, or lying belly-to-the-earth and letting Mumma Nature hold you. It might be wearing certain colours and fabrics – I won't lie, swishing around in my silky animal-print kaftans makes me feel like a total goddess.

What are some of the things that bring *you* sensorial pleasure? You might love a specific colour and the sensations that it evokes in you – right now I'm obsessed with a neon yellow and pink uplifting colour way – or you might really like the feeling of warm sand as you walk bare foot on the beach. Make a list. Get as descriptive as you possibly can, then put it up somewhere visible as a reminder of what makes you feel *goooooooood*.

My list includes:

——— the smell of first rain on sun-baked earth;

——— putting fresh linen on the bed – the sensation of climbing into delicious fresh sheets is EVERYTHING;

——— eating freshly picked juicy strawberries that I've grown myself, with love, from seed;

——— peonies and roses – so pretty;

——— dancing and sweating out my prayers;

——— eucalyptus and rosemary essential oils combined and used as a shower steamer;

——— the sound of waves crashing on the shore; and

——— the smell of my skin after a day at the beach – salty, sun-kissed and happy.

RECEPTIVITY AS A FEMININE SUPERPOWER

When our senses are alert, we are present, right here, right now, and we become much more open to receiving. Whether it's a compliment from your partner, the offer of help and support, an afternoon nap, a gift given with love or an uninterrupted night's sleep, receiving can be deeply difficult for many of us. We often feel like we have to 'give' (so that we can be seen as good) and 'do' (so that we can be seen as productive), and that the act of receiving is somehow passive, vulnerable, indulgent and/or lazy.

Not true.

Receptivity is a feminine superpower. Yep, instead of following the masculine/capitalist model of going out into the world, hustling, attention-seeking, being over-productive and often burning out in the process – when you're open to receive, you allow yourself to be met, exactly where you are. When I think of receptivity, I think of Cleopatra, laying on a chaise longue, simply being bloody glorious. She's just had a lovely luxe milk bath, she's put on her favourite ensemble, all the while whispering to herself: 'You are glorious, you are bountiful, you are powerful, you are whole.' She has enlivened all her senses and she's now open to receive.

Receptivity doesn't mean simply laying around waiting for something to happen, Cleo style. When you're connected to source and you're resourced, your sensorial nature is alert and you're able to really sense, meet, respond to and then tend to your own needs. And when you're not frantically doing, you're able to create space at your centre – and the stillness of that space becomes potent, because you're present. Fully present.

In fact, it's the very opposite of being weak and passive: when we're open to receive, we build a space bursting with a life-force and potential for creative power, thought and manifestation. When we nourish and tend to our own needs, when we allow ourselves to rest, dream, sleep well, eat well, move our bodies in delicious and sensual ways, drink the water, walk in nature and do more things that bring us joy and fewer things that create anxiety, this potent space of receptivity becomes magnetic, our reality aligns with our frequency and we become fecund and fertile – and in this place? Anything becomes possible.

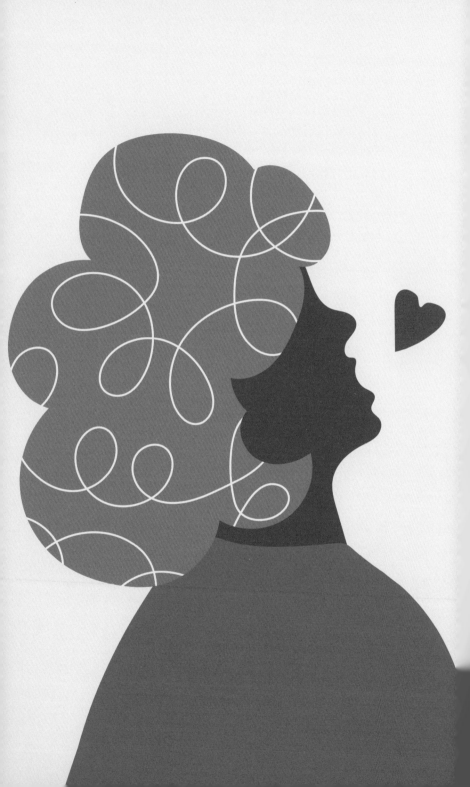

INVITATION:
HOLD AND TEND

When we talk of nurturing and tending to ourselves, it can activate big emotions and feelings, like *'I'm not good enough'*, *'I don't deserve it'* and *'It's selfish to put my needs before others'*. If you experience any of these, or your own version of similar thought patterns and programming, try this simple nurturing hold.

———

Place your fingertips on each side of your chest, aligned above your nipples, halfway between the tops of your shoulders and your nipples.

This hold nurtures and nourishes the body: it is a hold for self-nurturing, to mother yourself and to give yourself the big love.

This is often a tender spot for women, so be gentle. You do not need to press hard. Simply breathe deeply for several minutes, sending love and forgiveness through your fingertips and into your body.

SELF-LOVE IS A RADICAL ACT

To resource, tend to and nurture yourself in a world where women are taught that it's selfish or indulgent, or even narcissistic, to be top of their own priority list is actually really bloody radical.

Knowing what you want, desire and need (not what you're *told* you want, desire and need), and knowing how to source it, and that you deserve to fully receive it, breaks the spell. It breaks the chains of disempowerment. It breaks the demonising of the body and it reconnects you to your true nature as you reclaim your body and your life as your own.

It's you: vital, joy-filled, content, regulated, with self-set boundaries.

It's you: in your own body, connected, trusting and knowing that you are so worthy.

It's you: in alignment with your true-to-you frequency.

It's you: in constant communication with your present-state awareness.

MOON AND MENSTRUAL MAPPING

I've been sharing how to self-source for a few years now and, as with everything in this book, it's not a formula: it's a process of self-discovery and exploration. You do not need me to tell you to drink more water, move your body and eat less sugar. (Also, there's a whole ton of books and reading material online if that is the kind of information you're looking for.) This is different: it's an invitation to get curious. To become discerning about what we give our energy to.

How you get curious really is your call, but I'd love to share something that has changed my life. I call it Moon & Menstrual Mapping. Remember back in chapter 2, when I spoke about our connection to nature and our cycles as a way of understanding our emotional, spiritual and physical well-being? Well, that cyclic wisdom has also been the foundation of how I personally resource myself. I work with the phases of my menstrual cycle, but if you're not someone who bleeds, as I shared earlier, you can also use the cycles of the moon to explore this.

Working with the ebb and flow of the changing phases allows you to be connected to your ever-changing cyclical inner landscape: your emotional, physical and mental landscape. This helps you to recognise what you need in order to feel resourced, vital and fully alive in each phase.

My recommendation

I'll share a little bit about each phase so you have an idea of what might show up for you. Remember: everyone's wants and needs are different. I'll tell you what I've discovered I need in order to feel fully resourced and vital and in alignment with my frequency in that phase, and then, as you work with your own menstrual cycle or with the cycles of the moon, you can start to make notes and tune in to what *you* need in order to resource, nourish and nurture yourself in sync with *your* cyclic nature.

Pre-ovulation/Waxing moon

ENERGY: Masculine and outwards
SUPERPOWER: Being creative and taking risks

This is the phase in which to get work done, start new projects, go on dates, plant new seeds, try something new and basically take advantage of the renewed energy that's flowing through you. It's a powerful time to take a leap of faith, to take risks and make big changes in your life. Your productivity in this phase skyrockets.

Go get 'em, tiger!

To resource in the pre-ovulation/waxing moon phase:

———— I let myself think like a beginner.

———— I try things out and explore new things.

———— I diffuse jasmine oil, as it creates inspiration, passion and joy.

———— I go on morning jogs with sporadic breakout runs. My energy and hormone levels are beginning to rise after menstruation, so I actually like exercise in this phase – ha!

———— I schedule art dates with myself.

———— I let myself work more and rest less as I have the energy levels to get more done (knowing that, in the second half of my cycle, I rest more and work less!).

Ovulation/Full moon

ENERGY: Masculine and outwards
SUPERPOWER: Confidence and self-assurance

This phase is all about networking, showing up, expressing
your ideas and, more importantly, making them happen.
You're magnetic, self-assured and confident. In this phase,
you are capable of forging deep connections and making lasting
impressions. If you want to ask for a raise, give a presentation
or have a deep talk with your partner, this is the time to do it.

You are fire. Rarrrr!

To resource in the ovulation/full moon phase:

———— I schedule meetings and friend dates because I actually
     like to be around people in this phase – ha!

———— I listen to loud music and sing and dance my arse off.

———— I make out. Lots.

———— I fill the house with roses, wear rose perfume…
     and everything else to do with roses!

———— I use the masculine 'doing' energy to be super practical
     and get work done, answer emails, speak with colleagues
     and to do *all the things* (knowing that my energy levels
     will be lower as I move into the next phase).

Pre-menstruation/Waning moon

ENERGY: Feminine and inwards
SUPERPOWER: The ability to cut through bullshit

Often dreaded (mainly because most of us try to continue to keep 'doing' at the same pace we were in the first two phases of our cycle), this phase is potentially really powerful. It's a move into the feminine: an invitation to stop going so fast and doing so much and instead to turn inwards and be open to receive.

If you allow it, and don't resist it, this creates a lot of clarity. You may feel the need to clean, decorate or tidy the house, organise your office and filing system, and edit people and negative situations out of your life. Anything you've been sweeping under the carpet will reappear in this phase. You've been warned.

To resource in the pre-menstruation/waning moon phase:

———— I schedule fewer calls and meetings – my tongue is sharp and I'm without filter in this phase, so it's best for everyone.

———— I order a shit ton of cacao and either drink it as hot chocolate with coconut milk, honey and rose water, or nibble on a bar throughout the day. Either way, throughout this phase, my cacao consumption level is high.

———— I write sticky notes and memos to remind me that I'm a good person, because sometimes the inner critic in this phase is *loud*. I read these notes aloud to myself like affirmations.

———— I move my body in slow, sensual ways.

———— I use the expensive moisturiser and wear the expensive perfume.

Menstruation/Dark moon phase

ENERGY: Feminine and inwards
SUPERPOWER: Heightened senses and awareness of *everything*

This is *the* phase to connect with your inner wisdom. In fact, if you let it, this is an opportunity for deep reflection each month, a chance to release what's no longer necessary and relevant in your life and to really get a feel for what *is* necessary and relevant moving forwards. That way, you can plant the seeds for this as you move back in the pre-ovulation/waxing moon phase. Smart, huh?

To resource in the menstruation/dark moon phase:

——— If I have big decisions to make, I try to make them during this time. I often tell people – especially if they're asking me to make a big decision – 'Let me bleed on it'.

——— I limit calls or work meetings during the first few days of this phase.

——— I place my feet either in the dirt or in the sea if possible.

——— I use clary sage essential oil to soothe any cramps.

——— I say no.

——— I take naps.

——— I write my intentions for the cycle ahead – work, dreams, actual things that need to be done – so I don't feel overwhelmed going into the next cycle.

———

This is a super simple guide. This is how it is for me; it may not be how it is for you. What I need may not be what you need – so let yourself get curious. I share more insight on how to chart your phases and discover your superpowers through your cyclic wisdom in my book *Code Red: Know your flow, unlock your monthly superpowers and create a bloody amazing life. Period.*

GET CURIOUS

However you choose to explore your needs, wants and desires, let it be fun and playful. Let it be a process of self-kindness as you become aware of what it feels like to be a fully resourced human who is able to receive and not one who is constantly running on empty or feeling burned out.

If moon and menstrual mapping isn't your thing, as you breathe and connect with your heart and belly each morning, you might want to ask yourself the following questions:

——— Who and what do I need in my world in order to feel strong, stable and supported?
——— What kind of people nourish me?
——— What food makes me feel good?
——— What music or podcasts fill me up?
——— What movement and practices makes me feel vital and alive?

Take note of your answers and see if you can start to give yourself a little more of what you need (as well as paying attention to how you respond when you do so). Maybe you need half an hour a week to listen to your favourite podcast because you love learning from that particular presenter, and what they share supports you and makes you feel good. Give yourself that time. How does it feel? If any critical or judge-y voices show up, which they sometimes can when we start to nourish ourselves and give ourselves what we need, soothe them by telling them calmly, but with authority, exactly what's happening and that you deserve it. This may take a few goes, and you may feel the pull of something on your to-do list that seems far more important – but remember: *you* are important.

I DESERVE TO BE NOURISHED AND RESOURCED.

6: BE YOUR OWN AUTHORITY

(and your
top priority)

When life gets tough or challenging, it makes absolute sense that we would look to others for support and guidance. I pull a card from my SHE Sirens oracle deck daily, I'll often check in with astrology for the week ahead and I don't know what I'd do without my close counsel of favourite humans, the ones who I share and feel into all my 'stuff'with: they offer perspective, they share insight – and they've stopped me from spending way too much on a designer handbag (shit, it was pretty, though)! They also help me to be a lot kinder and nicer to myself than I sometimes feel capable of being, especially if I've messed up, and they call me out (with love) if I do or say something silly. (FYI: it's said that we're the average of the five people we spend most of our time with, so make sure the people you spend time with are the good ones. Hold them really close, treasure them and love them up. Hard.)

However, if you find yourself consistently deferring to other people, feeling like you absolutely, positively *need* the input of others in order to even begin to navigate decision-making, and thinking that someone always knows better than you and somehow has answers that you don't, then there's a chance that you're supressing your own inner knowing – that deep-belly wisdom that we spoke about earlier. By doing this, you hand over your agency and power and, in the process, diminish your presence.

YOU DON'T NEED TO BE SAVED.

NOT BY THE MYTHICAL KNIGHT IN SHINING ARMOUR, NOT BY THE GOVERNMENT, AND NOT BY THE LATEST SPIRITUAL WELLNESS GURU.

YOUR LIFE? *YOU* DECIDE

When we seek help or validation, it's usually because we want to do the 'right' thing, please people and not mess up, but guess what? There is no 'right' way. You absolutely cannot and will not please everyone all of the time, and, sometimes, you will mess up. It's inevitable.

No matter what you've been told or sold, no matter how much you try to live up to the 'good girl' archetype or try to please other people, you are the authority on your life. You get to decide what you wear, who you are in relationships with others, whether you adopt a cat, whether you eat the chocolate bar, what spiritual path you take, whether you accept that job... Yep. *It's your choice.*

Now, I'm not going to lie, it's much easier to not choose. Handing over the responsibility to someone else or asking a higher power or guru to 'take the wheel' is often way more appealing an idea than actually having to take responsibility and make your own choices. Thing is, so much of our societal programming relies on us thinking and believing we're powerless.

This is how it goes if we think we're powerless, we're less likely to create, we're less likely to have new ideas, we're less likely to want to be active participants in the creation and manifestation of our lives and reality, so instead, we become onlookers, sitting back and watching life happen to us.

Except – guess what? You are not powerless. That's the first – and most important –decision that you get to make: the decision to not accept the societal programming, the current reality, the story that you might have been told that somehow suggests you don't have power.

I have this quote, from Dr Clarissa Pinkola Estés, author of *Women Who Run With the Wolves*, taped up on my wall:

'As long as a woman believes she is powerless and/or is trained to not consciously register what she knows to be true, the feminine impulses and gifts of her psyche continue to be killed off.'

It's a reminder of all the times I have totally ignored my deep-down belly-knowing, my *inner-tuition*, and instead listened to others, the media, the societal 'shoulds', because I thought it was the 'right' thing to do. It's also a reminder of what happens as a consequence of doing this.

SELF-RESPONSIBILITY

Of course, we don't have *total* freedom, and there's inevitably some rules that we all have to abide by. I'm writing this during the 2020 pandemic. All around the world, people are having to stay in and not leave their homes due to a virus. It's an unprecedented situation, and yet everyone – from government officials to social media influencers – are telling us what we 'should' be thinking, doing and feeling, and how we 'should' be living in and experiencing this very surreal situation (in alignment with their perceived 'right' outcome, obvs). But the truth is, no one has the answer – whether we're talking about a pandemic or life in general. No one can truthfully say that their way is the *only* way (although, believe me, they will definitely try). So know this: even if you can't control or change a situation, you can choose how you see it, and how you respond to it. There are many realities running parallel with each other at any given moment, so many potential paths and possibilities open to us and, in every moment, *you* have the power to come into alignment with *your* frequency, what you know to be true to you, and choose to live *that* life.

Now, I know from personal experience that living a life in alignment with my values, tuned in to my frequency, involves me taking some serious self-responsibility for every decision and choice I make.

I'm not going to lie: self-responsibility can be uncomfortable. *Very* bloody uncomfortable.

But the pay-off?

Ohh, now that's juicy. *Very* juicy.

I AM A POWERFUL AND SOVEREIGN HUMAN.

INVITATION: DATE WITH DESTINY

Start by taking inventory. I know it sounds boring, and you may be tempted to skip this bit – but stick with me on this. It's so bloody helpful. Taking inventory isn't about passing judgement on yourself, your life or the decisions you've made in it. It's about knowing where you're at, so you can move forward with power and agency.

———

Make a date with yourself. Set aside at least an hour, make your favourite drink, bring some snacks and your journal and pen. To begin, take a few minutes to place one hand on your heart and the other on your belly. Bring your attention to your breath, align with your frequency and write down your answers to the following questions:

- What are your five from-the-core values?
- What do you stand for?
- What do you believe in?
- What lights a fire in your belly?

Now ask yourself (and note down) your response to: 'Are there any changes I need to make in my current life to come into alignment with these values and fire-starters?'

If you are currently living in total alignment and have absolutely no changes to make, high fives and fist bumps to you. I'm in awe.

If there *are* things to change, start by creating daily micro rituals and movements and working on just one thing at a time.

If you've recognised that you're a people pleaser – 'hi, nice to meet you, I'm Lisa and I'm a recovering people-pleaser too' – and that you give everything to everyone and do nothing for yourself, a daily micro-ritual might be to create ONE non-negotiable act that's only for you. Spend a half-hour reading a book in bed. Buy yourself flowers on a Friday (Venus day). Have a cup of tea and a morning stretch before the rest of the house gets up. Don't over complicate it; a micro-ritual is simply something that will honour you, support you to feel good and help you to stay in alignment with your values.

I carry out this practice every new moon – the new moon supports heart and belly-led intention setting – and for the most part, my responses remain the same. However, a regular check-in allows for fluidity and flexibility, and it helps me to stay vigilant to all the places where I may hand over my power, fall into 'pleaser' mode and become compliant because it's an 'easier' option than staying true and in alignment with myself. Don't get it twisted, it happens. Did I mention this wasn't a quick-fix formula? This is a process.

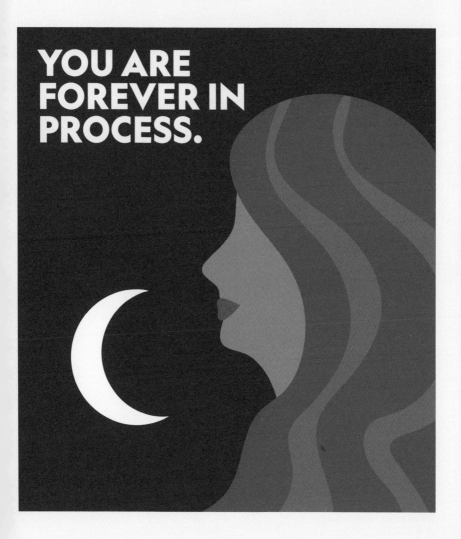

YOU ARE FOREVER IN PROCESS.

YOU ARE ENOUGH AND YOU ARE ENTITLED TO FEEL GOOD.

KNOW YOUR WORTH

*'When you say "Yes" to others, make sure you are
not saying "No" to yourself.'* – Paulo Coelho

Not so long ago, the idea of setting clear, non-negotiable
boundaries in alignment with my values and beliefs would have
had me running for the nearest available escape route. I would
rather have chewed at my own toenails than have to say no to
someone. I would have felt selfish and guilty, or I would have
stayed up all night going over and over exactly what I said and
how I said it, worrying that I might have hurt or upset someone.

Have you ever felt the same?

What I know now is that people will treat you exactly as you teach
them to – and how you teach them to treat you depends on how
'enough' you feel. If you have a deep love, respect and honour for
yourself, your self-worth will be high. You'll instinctively know what
is acceptable (and what is absolutely not acceptable), and you will
create the necessary boundaries required. If you talk negatively
to yourself, feel undeserving, guilt and shame yourself for things
you may or may not have done or if you have been taught that your
worth is dependent on how well you please and appease others,
your self-worth will be low, and setting boundaries will feel hard,
awkward and cringe-inducing.

Your self-worth is something *you* get to determine.

When you're aware of where in your life you're putting up with
things that you're not happy about, or simply tolerating and enduring
life rather than loving and enjoying it, you can see where you may
need to create strong and supportive boundaries. Just so you know:
you are entitled, and absolutely deserve, to feel good and to live
a life in alignment with your heart and gut wisdom.

SETTING BOUNDARIES

Setting healthy, non-negotiable boundaries and more importantly, keeping them, is a lived and learned practice that requires you to trust and believe in your most fulfilled, abundant vision for life.

Why do we need them?

Mostly so that that our own needs are not buried under a mountain of perceived, or real, obligation.

For me, setting boundaries used to feel difficult because I thought I'd disappoint people. Ugh, that's the worst. When I was a kid, if my mumma said she was disappointed in me, it was like a punch to my belly. With a bit of psychotherapeutic training, I've realised – and this is golden, so take note – people are disappointed when they have *any* kind of expectations as to who they want you to be and what they want you to do.

I know. It's a real truth bomb, isn't it?

If you're continually trying to meet the requirements necessary to live up to the expectations of others, then 1) it will be bloody exhausting, because 2) there are over seven and a half billion people on the planet and everyone has different expectations, so you will inevitably disappoint someone. You've heard that old adage, 'you can't please everyone all of the time', right? Never is it more true than when trying to meet other people's expectations of us – because they are exactly that: other people's expectations – their made-up version of us based on their thoughts, values and beliefs, not our own.

It might help to ask yourself: 'What's getting in the way of me setting clear boundaries for myself?' Are you worried people will think that you're rude, or perhaps that you're not a 'nice' or 'good' person? Maybe you're concerned that people simply won't like you?

'Your boundary need not be an angry electric fence that shocks those who touch it. It can be a consistent light around you that announces: "I will be treated sacredly."' – Jaiya John

Boundaries give you back your sense of power and agency over your experience. They state what your values are and how people can approach and communicate with you. They create a sense of safety for everyone. I used to really worry that people would think I was being aggressive or a bit angry for setting boundaries. I realise now that most people actually respond really well to clarity. Yep, the clearer I am about what is, and isn't, acceptable for me, the easier it is for people to respond and interact with me.

For example, if I'm invited to a party, and I'm premenstrual, I will give whoever has invited me the heads-up that I have limited energy and will only be attending the party for an hour. If that's not OK with them, I won't go at all. Simple.

In the same way, I won't take calls before 10 a.m. because I'm a morning person, and the time between 5.30 a.m. and 10 a.m. is *my* time. Sometimes I use that time to read, sometimes I write, sometimes I'll move my body, sometimes I'll chant. But honestly, *what* I'm doing is irrelevant. What matters is I will *not* talk to you before 10 a.m.

The more I practise setting boundaries that support how I live my life, the easier it becomes to express these boundaries to others clearly and without apology and to live a life that's mine, boldly, on my terms.

INVITATION: POWER CHARGE

If, for any reason, you're struggling to feel your power and to set boundaries that will support the choices you make in life, let this practice be a power surge to your system as you call back your power and autonomy.

—

Stand with your feet on the earth and your knees bent and soft.

Place both hands on the space about 5 cm (2 inches) below your navel.

Breathe deeply into the space beneath the palms of each hand. Do this for a few breaths, feeling present and in your body.

On the next inhale, breathe in and hold the breath deep in your belly, saying inwardly, 'I call back my power now'. Then, exhale, letting any resistance to the phrasing or the practice go with it.

Do this five times and, with each inhale, allow yourself to really feel your power and autonomy return to your body.

I CALL BACK MY POWER. NOW.

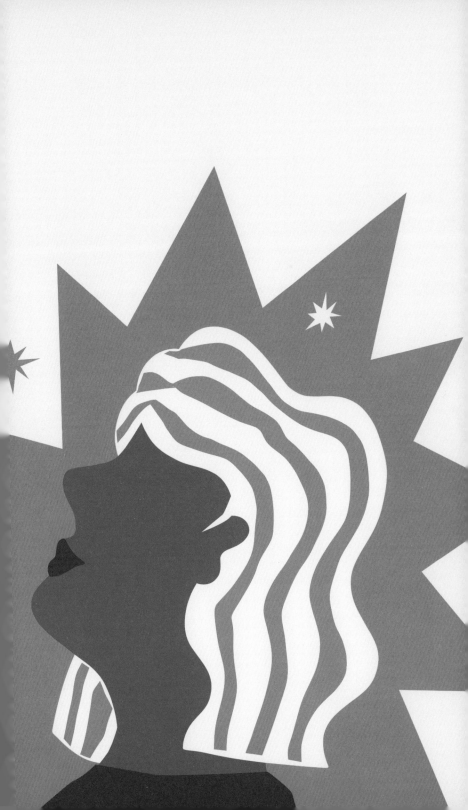

HELL YES, FUCK NO

There's a theory suggested by a dude called Derek Sivers, which essentially says that if you need to make a decision and your response is not a hell yes, then it's a fuck no.

Except most life decisions are a little more complex than that: there might be other people involved, there might be financial implications and, if we're not fully present in our bodies when we're making the decision, our *hell yes* or *fuck no* could be decided from a place of avoidance or destruction. Not good.

I mentioned in the previous chapter that if I have a big decision to make, I'll work with the phases of my menstrual cycle and I'll 'bleed on it'. I get how weird that might sound, and while it *has* been scientifically proven that women can make healthier decisions for themselves when they're menstruating, for me, it's mainly a super practical exercise in buying extra decision-making time.

I know my body well enough now to recognise her responses. If I have a decision to make, and my body response isn't juicy and warm and excited – that's what my *hell yes* feels like, by the way – then, ultimately, I know it's a *fuck no*. But it hasn't always been that way.

Many of us, women especially, have spent so much time modifying our *yes* and *no* to appease and to please that we've ignored our own internal bodily sensations.

If you've ever said yes when you meant to say no – and I have done this *far* more often than I'd like to admit – whether in the bedroom, in business, with friends or with family, just know that it was probably due to the deep survival programming that wants us to be liked and to stay safe in order to survive. Let's face it, it feels much safer to be seen and experienced as the 'yes girl' rather than the sovereign, resourced woman who feels, intuits, is IN her body and IN her power, doesn't it? But that safety is perceived. The real safety is found and felt when we honour ourselves, call back our power and trust our bodies.

Spoiler alert: you *do* know what you want.

INVITATION: ASK YOUR WHOLE BODY SYSTEM

If you have a big decision to make and you don't yet trust your *hell yes* and *fuck no*, try this exercise.

——

Begin by doing the Power Charge practice on page 116. Afterwards, allow yourself a few minutes to simply breathe, be still and be in your body.

Now place a hand on your heart and ask your question. *Feel* as well as listen to the response.

Place a hand on your belly and ask your question. *Feel* as well as listen to the response.

Finally, place a hand on your forehead and ask your question. *Feel* as well as listen to the response.

How did you feel and what, if anything, did you hear and/or see?

Some people will receive visuals, some people hear their *yes* or *no* as an actual voice, while others experience bodily sensations, such as chills, heat, shivers, heaviness or lightness. Take note of each response, then breathe deeply and let your entire body – your heart, gut and mind – respond to your question through your senses and know that, once you make a decision, it's the right decision.

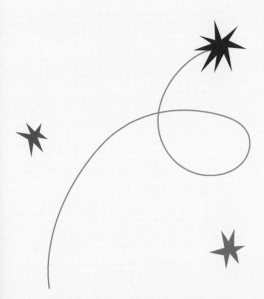

Look, trusting your body awareness won't make tough situations go away, and it doesn't mean that you'll never have to make another challenging choice ever again – you will – but when you tune in to your body, and recognise and read what your internal bodily sensations are trying to tell you, you build a trust and an understanding that it's OK to honour what your body wants.

FYI: It's OK to say 'no'

You can say 'no' with grace, without offending anyone and while staying completely in your power.
It *is* possible. I promise.

———— 'Thank you so much, but that doesn't work for me right now.'

———— 'I'm currently really busy, but I'm so grateful that you thought of me.'

———— 'It sounds great, but no thank you.'

———— 'No, I can't make it, but thanks for the invite.'

Alternatively, 'NO' is a complete sentence. Wink.

I HONOUR WHAT MY BODY WANTS.

I AM
A PRIORITY
IN MY
OWN LIFE.

BECOME YOUR OWN NUMBER-ONE PRIORITY

The only person responsible for making you feel worthy, cherished, loved, nourished, valued, happy and whole is *you*.

Don't let the responsibility of that become stress-inducing. (If it feels that way, check whether you're trying to live up to any unrealistic external references of the 'right' way to be you.) Instead, let this responsibility be a reminder of who you are, what you believe in, what you stand for, your personal power – and remember, when we're talking about power, we're talking about nourishing, creative power, not egocentric, controlling and competitive power. Let it be a reminder of how much better life is when your decisions about how to spend your time and energy are made based on your own frequency and inner wisdom, and not the validation and approval of others.

But here's a fun twist: the more you prioritise yourself, meet your own needs and align with your own frequency, the more magnetic you are, the more compelling you become, and the more compliments you'll get. Yep, the less you need that validation and approval, the more you'll receive.

My mantra? *I won't rely on compliments to feel good and worthy, but I will accept them with a big, open heart.*

———

NOTE: When I talk about self-trust and taking responsibility for yourself, please know that I'm aware of what a complex AND beautiful thing it is to cultivate. I get it. We've become so unaccustomed to finding the answers within that listening to our own voice can feel bloody dangerous. So, be patient with yourself. Yes, it might take time, it's a process, remember? Yes, you might still want to reach out to others for help – and if you ever feel like you're struggling, you should definitely do that – but returning to your body, taking responsibility for yourself, recognising you have power and agency over the decisions you make, the boundaries you set and how you choose to show up in your life is really powerful.

YOU ARE POWERFUL.

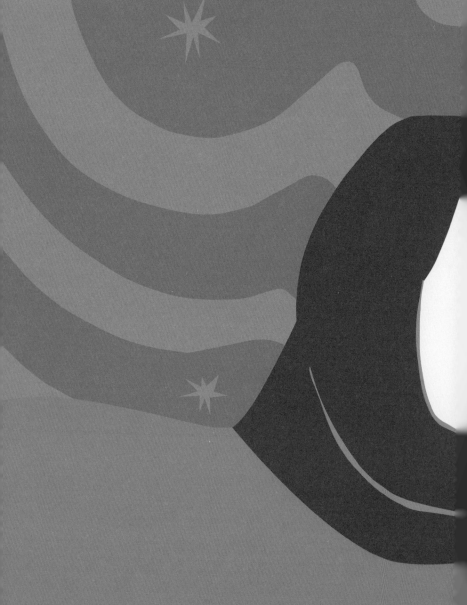

PART THREE: TAKE UP SPACE

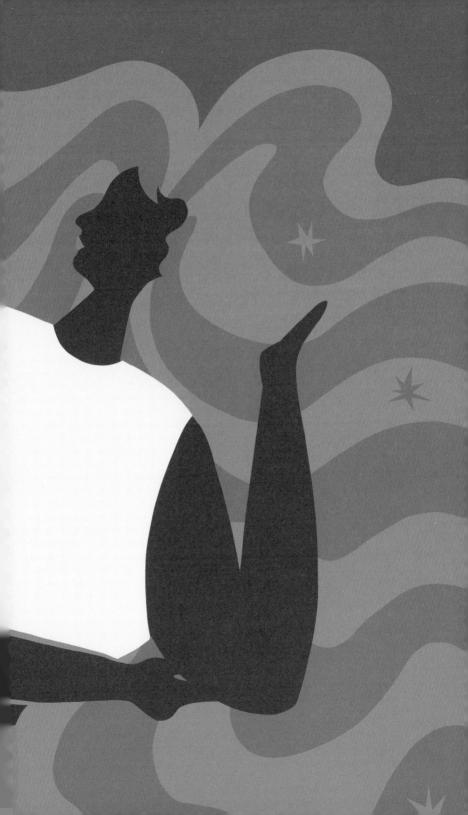

7: SHOW UP

You, expressed.
Fully.

I'm an introverted extrovert. It's a 'thing': you can Google it.

I like to be seen, I like to go to fun parties, I like to wear leopard print, I laugh really loud, I am a huge fan of a hot pink lip-and-nail combination *and* I also like to stay home, not talk to people, read a book, not turn my phone on for days, write words that people may or may not read and eat cake.

These are just some oversimplified, yet totally true and real contradictory expressions of me (there are many, many more). The amount of sleep I've had, who you are, what you want from me, where the moon is, how well I know you, how much I *like* you, how much energy I have and whether there's going to be food at the aforementioned fun party[3] are just some of the things that will determine the volume and expression of my presence.

I can say this now with no apology and zero guilt, because… yep, you've guessed it, *I know myself*. Back in the day, I was forever working against myself and my innate wisdom. I edited and censored how I expressed myself: the clothes I wore, the actions I took, what I said and how I said it. I was forever a 'version' of myself that I barely recognised.

[3] Horrifying, but true: there are some people who throw parties *without* food. They are *not* my people.

FEAR AND EXPOSURE

Why do so many of us *not* express ourselves fully?

Fear.

Never before has it been easier for us to have a voice, thanks to all the social media platforms at our disposal – yet sharing our truth, opinions and thoughts in the world can leave us feeling exposed, vulnerable and open to judgement, shaming and misinterpretation. In an interview with *Grazia*, chef and food writer Gizzi Erskine revealed that she sometimes censors what she says on social media, while Jameela Jamil shared the following Instagram post: 'When a woman steps up and speaks out, she's taken out of context [and] compulsively overexposed, her tone is exaggerated by media to look hysterical and violent, her integrity is questioned and society tries to slander her into silence. Every single time.'

Blame and shame are key players in the patriarchal playbook. They're weaved into our stories through social hypnosis, and used, really effectively, to manipulate people, especially women, into feeling, thinking, behaving and acting in certain ways. Nowhere is this more visible than on social media.

I'm not being a Debbie Downer, I promise. When we know how the cultural landscape is for so many of us, we can locate the source of 'fear', acknowledge it and then resource ourselves and cultivate what we need in order for us to be able to navigate it, take action and show up within it. Because no matter what, however we choose to do it, we *are* going to show up. (And we're going to really need to tap into all that compassion we cultivated back in chapter 1: both for ourselves, as we create the safe space we need to share our true expression; and also for others, including those – and this is the really bloody hard bit – that feel it's OK to shame, police, judge or call out someone else's thoughts or expressions.)

INVITATION: WHAT'S HOLDING YOU BACK?

Now, this one might feel a little ouch-y, and you may feel like you want to skip over it and move on to something that feels more fun. But if the idea of showing up has you feeling like an imposter, if your true expression feels stifled or if you're only ever sharing a watered-down version of yourself, it's time. We have to... *go there.*

Connect with your breath. Sit tall with the soles of your feet on the floor. Roll your shoulders back three times and lower your gaze.

Now ask your body the following questions:

- When do I bite my tongue and not say what I actually mean?

- Why is that?

- Do I do it more with certain people or in certain situations?

First, notice if there are any associated sensations that you feel when you ask yourself these questions. Locate them in your body and write down your answers. Once again, you're simply information-gathering, becoming curious about your experience. Ask yourself some more questions:

- Has there been a time when it's felt unsafe for me to be seen?

- Why was that?

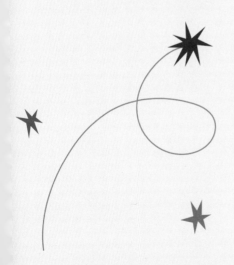

Again, feel the reactions in your body and then write down your responses.

Maybe you've experienced a confrontation in the past and vowed never to put yourself in that position again. Perhaps you were blamed for something you didn't do, publicly shamed for something you'd said or done, or accused of saying or doing something that had been misunderstood and totally taken out of context?

Whatever your experience, it's important to locate the reactions in your body, along with the stories and sensations that you've attached to them, and ask yourself: Is this story going to continue to stop me living a fully expressed life?

Now, please wrap your arms around yourself and give yourself a big hug. As you squeeze, locate the places in your body where those stories live and send the biggest love to them. Thank them for keeping you safe, and ask, as you release the hug, that they release their grip, even just a little bit, so that you can start to consider a different possibility. One where you are a glorious, fully expressed *you*.

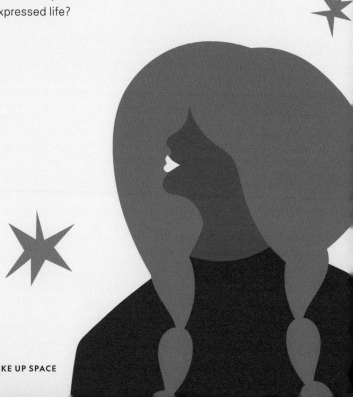

I AM WORTHY OF TAKING UP SPACE.

BEST SELF VS REAL SELF

So many of us are forever trying to be the 'best' version of ourselves, trying to brand ourselves as 'this' kind of person on our social media feeds, or 'that' type of go-getter in the office – but what if we dropped all that?

What if you dropped all the ways in which you've been *told* to show up? What if you stopped trying to be someone else's idea of what perfect/professional/good/right should look like and instead express who *you* are?

Your thoughts. *Your* art. *Your* dreams. *Your* words. *Your* energy.

Look, you don't have to pull a circa-1989 Madonna and 'Express Yourself' (although *do* watch the video, because honestly, Madonna is never *not* a schooling in true self-expression). You don't have to be an all-singing, all-dancing riot of colour, noise and energy in order to be yourself in your truest expression. That's totally *not* the point.

So what is the point?

In a world where you've been conditioned to be scared and fearful of being your true self, a world where you may have felt judged by others for expressing your truest nature, the point is this: to make every word, act and creation you share the most real and true expression of who you are, in that moment.

NO COMPARISON, LOTS OF COMPASSION

Now, this comes with a *massive* caveat. In life, and definitely on social media, people will always be keen to judge, to have an opinion, to tell you how you should show up.

And the truth is, we've probably all been judge-y of others, too, right? Comparing our experience with their on-screen highlights? I know I have. What I've realised is that comparison and competition will keep you in a state of fear and separation – and *that* will diminish your frequency and presence in the world.

So, let's stop policing and judging each other so harshly. We are ever-changing, messy and beautiful humans, which means our thoughts, opinions and expressions will be ever-changing, too. Let's allow there to be space for growth, for more than one reality, possibility and opinion. Let's agree to disagree; let's be open to changing our minds.

Please, for the love of all things fabulous, never let *anyone* tell you how to show up – and never tell anyone else how they should show up, either. *You*, on *your* terms, remember?

SHOWING UP IN THE WORLD IN A WAY THAT FEELS REAL AND RIGHT IS COURAGEOUS.

ALSO, IT'S ABSOLUTELY BLOODY NECESSARY.

FEEL THE REAL

Authenticity is another incredibly overused word, usually used by people trying to tell you how to be *more* authentic. Ha! That always feels really weird to me, because authenticity can't be taught by someone else or cultivated: it's *you*, revealed, uncovered, rediscovered and then fully celebrated.

What feels real to you will always bring power to your presence in a way that replicating the behaviour of others, putting on an act or being false could *never* do.

For some, feeling real will involve being deeply vulnerable and very open. For others it will involve being really private. Both are totally valid.

Responding to what feels real is a high five and deep bow of trust to your inner wisdom . FYI: Practising discernment in regard to what you choose to share and how you choose to share it in the world, whether that's in conversations with others or on social media, is not editing or censoring yourself; it's feeling into what feels real in that moment and responding (not reacting) accordingly. YOU get to choose, remember?

As with most things I've shared in this book, there's no one way to be authentic.

If you're present to what is, in alignment with the wholeness of who you are, all your parts, your presence is authentically powered. It's not about being the *best* version of you, or living 'your best life'; it's about having total agency over the choices you make, how you nourish and care for yourself, choose to spend your time and energy, and how you deprogramme, reprogramme and create your reality by continuing to choose YOU. Over and over again.

CREATE YOUR OWN REALITY

You are capable of actualising the biggest and boldest dreams and ideas that exist within you. It's why you're here. Which is great in theory, right? Yet another statement that would make a really good social media post. But *how* do you achieve it?

You own up to yourself about the big dreams.
You accept that you are worthy and deserving of good things.
You let yourself get stretchy with potential and you create space for... well, creation.

I'm from a council estate here in the UK and people like me were not taught to dream. In fact, it was actively discouraged. But, as you may have noticed, I've got really quite good at breaking the rules when it comes to doing what's expected of me. I've created my own rules and guess what? Someone like me is so worthy and deserving of ALL that she dares to dream of. Book deals, a hot Viking husband, a friend circle that is small yet mighty and who lift each other up (and eat cheese and laugh lots together), LA work residencies, people who love, support and buy my art and self-published oracle decks, clients and a community that I love and that I'm forever in awe of and inspired by, a little garden where I grow herbs, fruit and veg, and I've created a reality, my reality, that means I get to live a life in very close connection and communion with Mumma Earth and my own cyclic nature. People used to think it was radical, that it was so wildly different and 'out there' for me to approach life in this way – except it wasn't, not really. Basically, it just means I choose me. *Every time.*

I work for myself, I attract incredible clients and I do work that lights me up. I own my gifts and talents and share them in ways that feel good, real and expansive to me. I schedule my meetings, travel and appointments in a way that means I get to rest, work, create and play in accordance with my cyclic and rhythmic intelligence.

You can do this, too. You don't have to live life in total concordance to the moon or in alignment with your menstrual cycle (even though I totally, wholeheartedly, recommend it. I mean, I would, wouldn't I?), but when you know that you're not simply observing a pre-existing reality, you get to create your own adventure. It's not a 'manifesting' formula, it's a *knowing*.

YOU ARE THE CREATRIX OF YOUR REALITY.

YOU HAVE TWO CHOICES:

LET LIFE HAPPEN TO YOU

OR

CHOOSE TO MAKE MAGIC.

PLEASE CHOOSE TO MAKE MAGIC

A belly-deep knowing that says: you are worthy.

——— You are worthy of living a full, expressed life.

——— You are worthy of sharing that life with people and lovers who light you up and do not need you to perform in a certain way in order to make *them* happy.

——— You are worthy of doing work you love where you are paid well for your time, energy, wisdom and experience.

What's *your* reality?

Are you currently creating your own reality? Are the thoughts, opinions or expressions that you're having your own, or are they ones you're being told or fed, and are accepting as truth?

Creating your own reality involves you:

——— knowing who you are;

——— knowing what your values are;

——— staying tapped into your frequency and feelings as much as you can;

——— keeping your immune system strong; and

——— keeping your self-love high.

What choices can you make to take back command of *your* reality?

INVITATION: BECOME THE CREATRIX

When you choose to make magic, you accept that you're a creatrix and when you accept that you're a creatrix? ANYTHING IS POSSIBLE. Set aside half an hour for this practice.

———

Get comfortable and connect with your breath. As you read the following words, *feel* them move through your body.

Hold a fierce, technicolour vision for yourself of your life lived fully. Where are you? What are you doing? What does it feel like? Where can you feel it in your body? What sounds can you hear? Be as detailed as you can possibly be.

A life experienced through sensorial pleasure, through colour, sound and all that is vital. A life where you dance and hold court at the universal cosmic disco. (Yep, that's totally a place.)

Close your eyes, come down and into your body, and allow any colours, sensations, thoughts and dreams that come up to move through you.

Now dance, sing, rap, celebrate, speak, make art or shake your hips – whatever feels right to you – in response to that fierce technicolour vision. Allow it to live in and with you.

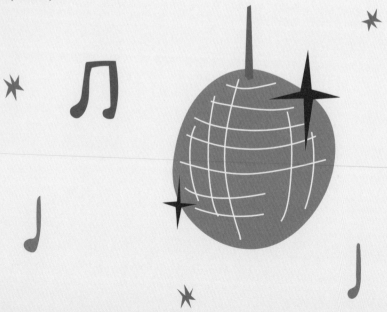

It's a mood. (Board.)

Anytime I do the creatrix practice, I respond to my fierce technicolour vision by creating a mood board. If I'm writing a book, I'll create a mood board for it. If I'm calling in a love, I'll create a mood board for it. (Yep, there was definitely a mood board made to call in my hot Viking husband.) The act of cutting up pictures, finding the right words and colours and images and sticking them together to support my vision is so helpful to me (it's a throwback to my 'zine making days in the 90s – remember *those*?). People fall in and out of love with the idea of mood boards and vision boards, but I have so much proof that they help bring my dreams and visions to life that I can't *not* mention them. If old-school cutting and pasting isn't your jam, write your vision into being through poetry or a song, sing it out loud or turn it into a dance that you do daily.

MAKE YOUR OWN KIND OF MUSIC

Your creative expression doesn't care what someone else 'thinks'. It doesn't care if it looks or sounds 'right'; it doesn't care if it's going to mess with how comfy you may or may not feel. Your creative expression is the forever-present fire in your belly, the impulse that wants, more than anything, for you to stop living in fear and instead to live in daily devotion to your values, your feelings, your gifts and your talents by expressing them so that they're seen, heard and witnessed.

A life lived without healthily expressing yourself – your anger, your sadness, your joy, your art, your thoughts, your opinions, your song, your truth, your gifts and your talents – will cause you pain mentally, psychologically and physically. But know this: if you're currently living an unexpressed life, you do have the capacity – and, more importantly, the courage, deep down inside of you – to turn that pain into power.

My poetic love was, is, and forever will be, Rumi. He gave up all his swanky educational titles and achievements to become a devotional dervish Sufi master. Swoon. I love a dude that's willing to go against the grain for what he believes in. Hot, right?

His words continue to speak straight to the heart of anyone who hears or reads them, even now, centuries later. He once said: 'Your task is not to seek for love, but merely to seek and find all the barriers within yourself that you have built against it.' Basically, he believed your *only* duty as a human is to recognise what wants to be expressed through you, and then remove all the obstacles that stand in the way of you expressing it.

So, be willing to:

——— be 'different' to how others might expect or accept you to be;
——— stop trying to be 'good' and 'right';
——— be heard; and
——— dare to take up space with your voice, your words, your dreams and ideals.

A fully-expressed human is my favourite kind of human. We are the game-changers and paradigm shifters.

Now, for some, that fullest expression will look like activism. For some, it will be writing books, making music or creating art. For some, it will be fierce self-sourcing. For some, it will be exploring new ways to heal. For some, it will be bringing children into the world, supported and loved. For some, it will be… well, you get the idea.

There's a gazillion options and possibilities, but just so you know, *you*, in your fullest expression, are not only *needed* in these 'interesting' times: you're bloody necessary.

(No pressure, obvs.)

8: OWN IT

Know what
you want and
how to get it

Often, for many, many reasons, we choose to play small.
We choose to stay quiet and not be seen. We shrink ourselves,
both physically and metaphorically, so that we don't attract attention,
so that we don't offend anyone, so that we don't take up space.

Why?

Because it can feel really bloody risky just to *be* who we are.

Whether we're trying to hide what we perceive as, or have been
told are, our dark and gnarly parts that we 'should' feel guilty or
shame about, or we're playing down our glorious and powerful
parts because we don't want to be seen as 'tooting our own horn'
or a 'show off', we do this because it feels like there's a possibility
– a really strong one – that sharing exactly who we are and what
we're *actually* feeling will mean we'll be judged, abandoned
and/or rejected.

Surely, it's waaaay safer to curate a palatable, easy-to-consume
version of yourself, one that ensures you avoid conflict, judgement,
put-downs and rejection? Right?

Yes, it might be safer, and you might avoid *some* conflict.
But in doing that, you will also miss out on a gazillion possible
opportunities to be surprised, annoyed, loved on, met by and
understood (and misunderstood) by other humans.

A gazillion possible opportunities to learn, grow, connect and
expand as a human.

A gazillion possible opportunities to experience a life fully lived.

WHAT WOULD IT BE LIKE TO OWN IT?

What would it be like to honour, acknowledge and even, dare I say it, *love* yourself? And I mean *all* of yourself: your tendencies, your quirks, your skills and talents, your secrets, your mess-ups and mistakes, your desires, your fears, your anxiety *and* your neuroses. What would that be like?

What if your default setting *wasn't* to shut parts of yourself down or off entirely, or to go along with something that someone else says so you remain 'likeable'? What if, instead, you recognised that all your parts make up the whole, that they *all* make you who you are? What if you make no apology for who you are, and instead, declare 'I am me and I am powerful, fabulous, brilliant, smart...'? (Add your own term of declaration here.)

Now *that's* a power move.

One that changes *everything*.

But no matter what self-help books or social media will have you believe, as we're exploring in this book, it's not a simple, click-your-heels-together-three-times situation.

Slowly and surely, with daily repetition, you start to find reflections of your declarations in your actions and the ways that others respond to you and the declaration becomes rooted in truth.

DON'T MEASURE YOUR PROGRESS WITH SOMEONE ELSE'S RULER.

UNREALISED POTENTIAL

Do you know the main reason we get jealous, envious and compare ourselves to other people?

Unrealised potential.

Yep, if you're not having great sex because you're too scared to ask for what you really want in your relationship, there's a good chance that someone who is having epic sessions in the bedroom (and the living room, and the kitchen) will make you jealous.

If you don't have love (or even like) and acceptance for your body, there's a good chance that someone who shares a picture of themselves with the caption 'looking cute' and gets 1,000 likes for it on social media will make you jealous.

If you're not doing work you really love, and you see someone who is unashamedly and proudly doing what they love in the world, sharing their passions *and* making money from it, there's a chance they will make you jealous.

For the most part (there are a few exceptions, but not many), when you find yourself comparing your life with someone else's, it's usually a sign that there is potential within you, currently lying dormant, that is desperate to be realised, owned, loved on, expressed and celebrated.

When I'm 'activated' (that's my nice way of saying 'When something or someone on social media is triggering the shit out of me'), it's usually because someone is actualising and claiming a desire that... well, I'm not.

We all know that social media is only a teeny, tiny showreel of what that person is actually doing, living and experiencing, but that does not always stop the comparison klaxon from sounding.

For me it sounds the loudest when:

— I'm writing a book and someone else makes the act of book-writing seem really glamourous and easy. Grr.

— I'm in the UK, it's raining, I'm wearing baggy tracksuit bottoms and someone shares how they've landed a three-month contract working in the sunshine doing something thoroughly fabulous. Grr.

— Someone has their shit together. This isn't just on social media – it happens if I see someone's got mad organisation skills, if they're always on time, if their bookshelves are organised by colour, if they remember to take tote bags every time they go to the supermarket. Grrr.

Weirdly, though – and stay with me on this one – feeling a sense of comparison can actually be a good thing. Yep, while feeling 'activated' can definitely be uncomfortable, chances are that the klaxon is sounding to let you know what exactly is waiting and wanting to be realised, actualised and claimed within *you*. It's not actually about the other person at all.

INVITATION: 'ACTIVATE' YOUR CURIOSITY

Don't just wait until you get 'activated' by something. If you do, this exercise will become a lot harder to complete. Instead, take some time to connect to your breath. Sit comfortably with your feet on the floor and set a timer for 20 minutes max.

———

Now, ask yourself the following questions:

- When do I feel envy, jealousy and/or comparison the most?

- Are there any particular people or situations that make me feel this way?

- What is it exactly about this person/situation that has me feeling like that?

- Be honest now – what is it about this person/situation that I want/require/desire?

- What's stopping me from making it true for me, too?

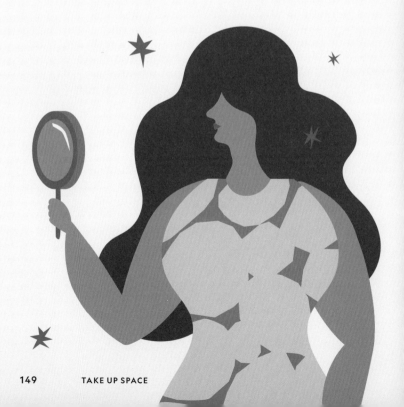

NOTE: This is *not*, I repeat, this is *not* an opportunity to beat yourself up for not having the 'thing' or not doing the 'thing'. It's designed to help you understand why you're feeling what you're feeling, a chance to make an honest assessment so that you don't stay stuck. If we stay stuck in comparison, it can be debilitating. We do nothing except get *more* angry and *more* resentful, which creates excess cortisol (the stress hormone) in the body, which then builds resentment and continues to keep us in the comparison loop. Not good. This exercise is about encouraging you to recognise, own and celebrate your unrealised potential. Just know that, if you're feeling envy, jealousy and comparison in your body, these feelings are a signpost to what wants to be realised or celebrated within you. Every day is a school day when it comes to learning more about the magic unfolding of YOU.

FORGIVENESS AND THE SHADOWS OF SHAME AND BLAME

Look, we've all made decisions in our lives that have been less than stellar, right? And yes, we may have harmed ourselves or harmed others in the process, but please, let what I'm about to say land in your big, beautiful heart: it is NORMAL human experience to make mistakes, to have errors of judgement, to mess up.

However, when we allow that shame and blame to persistently reside within us, it retreats to the shadows and can become heavy, dense and all-consuming, where it works predominantly to keep us small, keep us in fear and keep us from shining our light.

We all have shadows. If we shut down and deny them, it can become really tricky for us to recognise and course-correct when things may need to change. If we live them as our truth, we disconnect from our intuitive heart and belly wisdom, we don't trust ourselves to make decisions and instead, we allow ourselves to be led by our fear.

Neither is ideal for optimal life-living.

Rather than feeling bad or ashamed, shutting down or beating ourselves up for mistakes we may or may not have made, it is far more beneficial to our health and wellness to shine light into those dark places, to let it all be seen and witnessed and to use the shadow as an opportunity for reflection, to learn, grow, develop and show up in our wholeness. If you're feeling envy, jealousy and comparison in your body, these feelings will be a signpost to what wants to be realised, changed up or celebrated within you.

DON'T TRY TO MAKE PEOPLE LIKE YOU.

LIKE YOURSELF.

SELF-RESPONSIBILITY

When you dare to get curious (and honest) – whether it's about the places you experience comparison, or because you've upset someone, where you experience shame or because you think or feel a certain way about a person or a situation – you create space (and the courage) to ask: 'What's *actually* going on here?'

You create space to see what *might* be being projected on to you because someone else is scared, or because the TV show you're watching has an agenda, or because you and your true-to-you frequency make someone feel uncomfortable.

You create space for the possibility that you *might* have messed up; that your opinion or belief *might* be wrong. (Know that it takes practice and really *big* courage to create the space for this one, but the pay-off of acknowledging when you mess up and then taking action to course-correct is *gold*.)

You create space to recognise what's yours and what isn't. You don't pass the buck, you don't avoid the uncomfy feelings or conversations, but you also don't accept what's not yours to process or take responsibility for.

When you do that, when you own what's playing out for you (based on what you know and feel to be true for you), the energetic and emotional 'charge' is released. (Or lessened at least.)

You recognise that the way you're feeling is rarely about the actual person or situation you're faced with. You see and understand what needs to be accepted and/or changed, and then, and this is the good part, for the sake of the planet and all humanity, there's a capacity for compassion and forgiveness, both for yourself and for others.

Self-responsibility = self-power.

NOTE: While you're doing this discovering, unlearning and relearning, it's important that you take care of your heart, your mind and your nervous system.

Don't hide – and don't apologise (unless you're being a dick)

Ways to help make sure you're being true-to-you *and* not being a dick include:

——— Taking responsibility for learning about yourself *and* the world around you.

——— Recognising that you're not always right.

——— Letting go of unrealistic attempts to be perfect.

——— Being open to other people's opinions and recognising that you can still be friends with people that have differing views and opinions.

——— Becoming a 'felt' and belly-wisdom-led intuitive thinker.

——— Knowing that you don't have to stand down just because someone's shouting louder than you.

——— Having both passion and compassion.

——— Speaking about and expressing the things that are important to you.

There's no doubt that it takes courage and guts to own who you are, what you want, what you stand for and what you have to offer the world – yet doing this is how your presence truly becomes your power.

One of my favourite artists, Georgia O' Keeffe, said: '*I have already settled it for myself, so flattery and criticism go down the same drain and I am quite free.*' When you don't change yourself to try and be 'less threatening' or to try and fit in, be seen as 'acceptable' or to try and get others to fall in love with you; when you take responsibility for your actions; when you dare to dance with your shadows – you become free.

And that freedom is where a *real* sense of safety comes from.

You know yourself and all your parts so intimately that no one can ever 'have' anything on or over you. No one can blame you, shame you or make you feel less-than.

You can become integrated, embodied, all-in.

You get to like, love and respect yourself, know your worth and own who you are.

You're present and you're whole.

9: IGNITE YOUR LIGHT

How to magnetise,
radiate and be seen

If being present and whole is the 'goal', then what's next?

What do you *do* with that?

You ignite your light and you shine. BRIGHT.

You let your presence vibrate at your true-to-you frequency and you become a lit torch that shines so bright you are a radiant beacon of love, power and possibility.

There's nothing to *do* here.

No pushing, striving, hustling, or looking for the approval of others.

You're in your body. You're connected to source and you're resourced.

Your heart is open, you're centred at your belly.

Your breath is easy and in sync with your rhythmic intelligence.

You're grounded, you can feel Mumma Earth beneath your feet and you know that wherever YOU are is sacred ground.

You're aware both of yourself and of those you're in connection with, noticing energy, feelings, sensations, details and nuances.

You don't react. (At least not ALL the time – we're forever in process, remember?)

You practise discernment. You pause, you *feel*, you respond.

This is you, present and powerful.

THE POWER OF BEING SEEN AND HEARD

Are you scared of being powerful?

I'd totally understand if you were, because we often mistake the idea of power and what it means for the out-of-date patriarchal kind of power we've seen demonstrated by *some* men in positions of authority, or the 1980s shoulder-padded, green-eyeshadow-wearing, 'I-will-step-on-you-and-crush-you-in-order-to-get-to-the-top' kind of power we may have seen demonstrated by *some* women in the workplace. (These are extreme stereotypes, but you get the idea, right?) Our fear of what we perceive power to be and mean can have a direct impact on how much we want to be 'seen' in the world.

———— Do you like to be seen?
———— Do you like to be the centre of attention?
———— Do you speak up about things that
you believe are wrong or unjust?
———— Or do you prefer to be out of sight
and behind the scenes?

There's nothing wrong with any of these being your preference – as long as it actually *is* your preference. If, though, you're being loud as an act of bravado, or you're being quiet because you don't want to rock the boat, then you're not being fully present to *your* presence. Being present to your presence isn't always easy. We've been led to believe that those who like to be the centre of attention or speak loudly and proudly are 'too much', while those that like to be out of sight or aren't speaking up are 'not enough'.

It can seem like a no-win situation.

Often, as a woman, I've been told to 'shhh' and be quiet. As a woman in a bigger body, I've been accused of taking up too much space. I've been told to lose weight and be less than I am. As a woman who likes to wear a hot pink lip, leopard print dresses and flowers in my hair, I've been accused of drawing too much attention to myself.

When I didn't know better, when I heard these comments, I'd shrink to fit. I'd diet, I'd dim my light, I'd be more accommodating and do what I could to stay on the 'right' side of societal norms.

Now?

Now I call BULLSHIT. Really loudly.

However you choose to show up in the world is absolutely up to you.

You get to declare, on a daily basis: 'This is what I know and feel, deep down in my belly, to be true, right now.'

Imagine that. *You* get to set yourself free, put yourself at the centre of your experience, make up your own mind and fully express yourself.

Fully sovereign. Fully in your power.

YOU DON'T NEED ANYONE TO GIVE YOU PERMISSION TO BE YOU.

INVITATION: POWERFUL PERSONAL PRESENCE

When we have a powerful personal presence (yes, yes, I love an alliteration), we are comfortable with being seen and heard in ways that are in total alignment with the truth of who we are. We fully inhabit our being, trust our deep-belly wisdom and we are able to take up space without apology or approval.

———

This is a simple practice to build your energy so that you can *feel* yourself in your body and in your personal power. (I do it before workshops or meetings, but you can make it part of your morning practice – and, if you get to be in the sunshine, expand in the direction of the sun. Let the light really fill you up.)

Stand with your feet firmly on the floor. Bend at the knees, with your arms by your sides and bring your focus to your centre, to that space just below your navel.

Connect with your breath.

Feel steady at your core. Feel the earth beneath the soles of your feet.

Now, inhale deeply, in through the nose and into the chest and belly. Pause, then exhale through the nose. Keep going.

As you fill your chest with air, feel your body expand and stretch upwards and outwards. Feel your shoulders roll back, your neck lengthen, your spine straighten, your chin begin to raise.

Feel your arms outstretch, widening away from your body, stretching your personal space. Let your palms and fingers stretch wide, too, in order to create even more space.

Feel yourself anchored and strong in your navel space.

Feel your chest expand with each inhalation.

Stay in this position for anywhere between one minute to five. Keep your arms strong. Let the warmth build in your body, feel the sensations and keep the breaths coming in and out long through the nose.

When complete, let your arms drop to your sides and allow your breath to return to its usual pace. Be present for a few moments so you can really *feel* your powerful personal presence. It's not an identity, it's a felt force, and you get to choose how you share it in the world.

LIGHT YOURSELF UP

When we consciously feel our powerful personal presence as
energy and sensation in our body, we know it exists, we know we
exist and we can light ourselves up from the inside out with joy,
passion, devotion, play and love.

What lights a fire in your belly?

When you focus your energy on what fills you up, what lights you
up, what satiates you and most importantly, what feels really bloody
good? YOU are no longer disconnected, scattered and dissipated.
The process of reciprocation is juicy, vital and nourishing. You never
get worn out or tired: you're sourced by source energy itself and it
feels GOOD.

If I ever find myself wondering 'What's this life all about? What's
the point?' (which I sometimes do, because, y'know, I'm human),
I refer to my light-me-up list. A list I keep in the front of my journal
that includes people, quotes, music – anything or anyone that
creates fire, love and light in my belly. It also acts as a devotional
gratitude altar to all that I include on the list too like Salt 'n Pepa
(and let's not forget Spinderella) for my forever favourite album
Hot, Cool & Vicious, Paris for being the city where I have done a
lot of my most favourite kissing (it's also where my Viking husband
proposed to me – I know, cute, right?) and Hilma af Klint – another
artist I love who was way ahead of her time. Being in reverence
and thankfulness to the things that make you feel good amplifies
the 'feel good', so you're then able to let more in, and, to be clear,
we want to let as much feel good in as possible!

YOU'RE *ALLOWED* TO BE HAPPY

Writing a light-me-up list, letting light and joy in, being grateful to it so you can let even more in, is not as easy as it sounds. For many of us, me included, despite endlessly seeking joy, we daren't let it in. We've tried so bloody hard to control our experiences, to keep ourselves safe by doing the 'right' thing, that we've forgotten how potent and powerful joy, light, love and happiness actually is.

For most of my life, I held a strong cynicism for the whole 'light, love, blessings and gratitude' situation. I admit it, I have often given people who seem to be genuinely joyful the side eye.

What's that? Write down three things you're grateful for? Pah. No thank you. Why? Well, lots of reasons, all of which I know now were based in fear-filled, 'poor me' stories that led to me creating a protective armour of snark and sarcasm that actively cock-blocked All. The. Good. Things.

Now, while I believe that healthy questioning of everything should be encouraged, it doesn't have to come at the expense of allowing yourself to experiment with the 'lighter' side of life; to experience joy, fun, laughter, play and pleasure.

I now know and, more importantly, experience in my being that the more grateful I am for what I have, the more blessings I am able to receive. The more pleasure and laughter I allow myself to experience, the bigger my capacity to call in even more.

FYI: I still believe that the term 'love and light' is thoroughly over-used, though. Just saying. Wink.

You're allowed to be happy.

Yes, we're experiencing and navigating 'interesting' times; yes, there's death and destruction in the world. But allowing yourself to be consumed by it, to react to every news story, to throw yourself into every campaign is the sure-fire route to burnout.

We need you light-filled, we need you resourced and open to receive and claim your blessings, we need your powerful presence. That way, you're a safe space, someone that not only you trust, but who others can trust, too. Whether you stand on a stage, work in a supermarket, are a front-line activist, care for an elderly relative, campaign for animal rights or write a *New York Times* bestseller, that is how you can create impact and change in the world.

'Claim your blessings.' – Zen Nest

HOW MUCH JOY AND PLEASURE CAN YOU HOLD?

Very few of us have been taught how to let joy and pleasure be present in our being for more than a fleeting moment without swiping it away or playing it down, or feeling like we don't deserve it, so my invitation is to s-l-o-w-l-y expand your capacity to let in and to hold on to both joy and pleasure.

I make a playlist of five or six songs that make me feel glorious and evoke pleasure, joy and sensuality within me. I set a clear intention: *for 20 minutes, let joy, pleasure and happiness be present in my body.* Then I hit play. That's it. I create a space where I feel safe to dance, shake, move my body, without inhibition. I feel my toes, stamp my feet, stroke my hair, tap my body, move my hips (if you make no other movement, bring attention to your hips – they hold precious medicine, stir it up). I don't try to control any sensation of joy or pleasure or sounds I might want to make. Instead, I pay attention to my breath and I see if it's possible to expand those sensations throughout my whole body.

The trick is not to tense or tighten (although if you have a tendency, like me, to want to control ALL THE THINGS, this will take a little practice and patience) and instead to keep expanding the possibility that your body can hold joy. You can practice this during sex, too – either with yourself or with a partner – if it feels safe and good to do so. What you're looking to do is hold that joy and pleasure and all the sensations that go along with it IN your body. To let it all be present, instead of releasing it quick and fast, or constricting and controlling the pleasure, or getting overwhelmed because you don't think you can handle it. You can. Handle it, that is.

You have the capacity to hold so much joy, happiness and light. Allow the joy and happiness to meet your edges, to stay, until any excess joy fizzes to the surface and then, well... let it be FULLY experienced. Wink.

YOUR WHOLE SELF IS WELCOME HERE.

INVITATION: SOFTEN TO OVERWHELM

Now, while we're exploring and experimenting with how much joy we can hold, if it really *does* get overwhelming – and sometimes it can – this exercise can help you to soften.

———

Pull out a rug, or if you're able to, go outside and lie on Mumma Earth. Lie on your front and turn your head to the left side. Place your palms flat on the floor.

Breathe deeply.

Feel yourself belly to belly with Mumma Earth and soften.

Let your weight drop into her.

Soften your gaze. Soften your lips. Soften your tongue. Soften your face. Soften your jaw.

Soften the back of your head. Soften your neck. Soften your shoulders.

Soften your arms, your elbows, your wrists, your palms, the backs of your hands and your fingers. Soften your back body, your front body, your left-side body, your right-side body. Soften your belly. Soften your hips. Soften your buttocks. Soften your sexual organs. Soften your thighs. Soften your knees. Soften your shins. Soften your calves. Soften your ankles. Soften the soles of your feet, the top of each foot and your toes.

Let yourself be soft.

Feel Mumma Earth below you.

She's got you. She can hold you. She can hold it all. Let her show you how.

Lie there until the energetic charge and feeling of overwhelm lessens, and you return to centre.

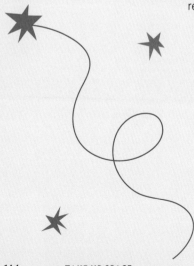

WHAT THE WORLD NEEDS NOW IS… MORE *YOU*

In a world that is becoming increasingly fragmented, inflamed, complicated and complex, there is so much for us to hold in our awareness right now – so many causes to support, so much to stand for, so much injustice to stand against – that the work, the ever-unfolding, ongoing process of being you, is to remain present to the power of your presence and allow your presence to stay present to it all: to stay present to yourself and your inner landscape, while engaging with, and tending to, the outer needs and requirements of your life, the people you love and care about, and the world you live in.

This, like everything I've shared in this book, is a practice.

As you reconnect with yourself, your body and your wisdom, you reconnect with others, you reconnect with nature and you reconnect with the planet. As you continue to learn, expand, heal and reveal, you become stronger, your heart and capacity for kindness expand, and you care more. Not only for yourself, but also for your family, for those you love, for your communities and for the world that you live in.

When you're full up, lit up and trust your own authority, you're able to be of service in a way that doesn't deplete you or burn you out because you're not reacting to life – you're responding to it.

You're able to fully witness, own and respect your strengths, gifts, connections, talents, knowledge, power and resources, and you're able to ask yourself: 'How can I use these to support and be of service to others?'

You don't try to fix the entire world all at once because you know that's simply not possible. Instead, you work to support and heal the parts that you are able to reach. Not by schooling people, preaching to them or telling them what to do. Instead, it is through your presence – the actions you take and the expressions you make from your place of wisdom, love and power as an in-your-body human – that you have the biggest influence, and it's powerful.

Really bloody powerful.

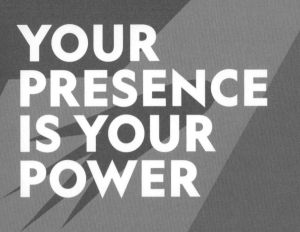

YOUR
PRESENCE
IS YOUR
POWER

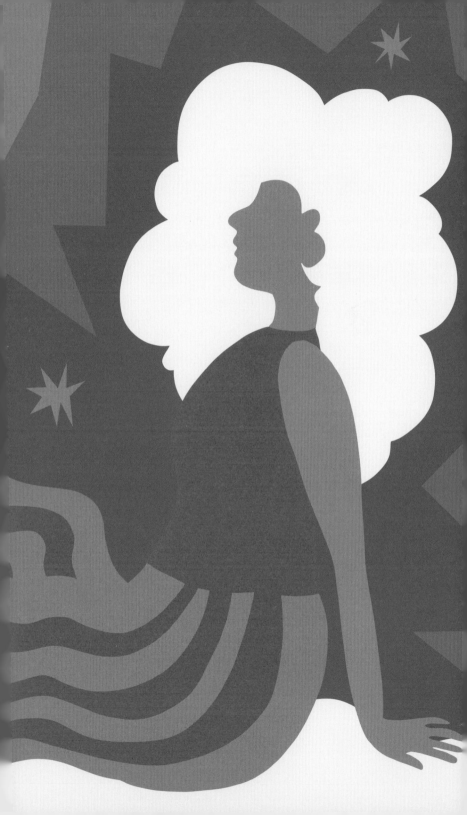

YOU ARE
POWERFUL

You have let go of who you thought you were
and who you were told to be, and instead fully
embrace and love on who you are.
You are powerful.

You know that what other people think
of you does not define you.
You are powerful.

You have set yourself free from any judgement.
You are powerful.

You know you are worthy and beautiful,
not because others think and tell you so,
but because you've decided to believe it's true.
You are powerful.

You stay true to your feelings, opinions,
thoughts and emotions (and also check in
with them daily, because you're open and
you know that you may change your mind).
You are powerful.

You have stopped explaining yourself,
what you want and who you are.
You are powerful.

You live your life, on your own terms, with
no apologies (unless you're being a dick).
You are powerful.

You are proudly present to the power
of your own presence.
You are powerful.

AND FINALLY...

In case you need
a reminder, your presence
is your power. Fill this
page in, rip it out, place
it someplace where
you'll see it daily.

———

WHEN WAS I BRAVE AND COURAGEOUS?

WHAT AM I MOST PROUD OF?

WHO DO I STAND FOR AND SUPPORT?

WHO HAS MY BACK?

WHAT LIGHTS ME UP?

WHAT ARE MY SUPERPOWERS?

WHAT IS MY SELF-DECLARATION
OF POWER AND PRESENCE?

You, in your fullest expression – not hiding, not self-editing, not keeping parts of you that you feel worried won't be accepted or that you think you will be shamed for pushed down or out of sight – you are powerful.

You are fierce fire and light.

A beacon of hope and magic in these 'interesting' times.

You don't need permission.

You don't need validation.

You don't need acknowledgement.

You are your own permission slip.

You validate your own actions, pat your own back and declare yourself a fierce and necessary powerful presence in the world.

ABOUT
THE AUTHOR

Lisa Lister is a bestselling author, artist, well woman therapist and a yoga and somatic movement teacher. She offers practical, psychological and spiritual tools, guidance and support to women who are exploring, navigating and healing their relationship with their body, their cycles, their sexuality and their power.

www.thesassyshe.com

INDEX